Pathology A to Z

- a Handbook for Massage Therapists

Pathology A to Z
- a Handbook for Massage Therapists

Kalyani Premkumar MBBS MD CMT

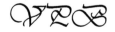

VanPub Books
Calgary - Canada

Notice to Reader:
This publication is intended as a reference book only, not as a medical manual. The information imparted is to help you make informed decisions in the practice of massage therapy. It will be prudent to seek medical advice, when in doubt.

Copyright © 1996 Kalyani Premkumar

ISBN 0-9680730-0-X

Published by
VanPub Books
Banker's Hall, Box No. 22325, Calgary, AB T2P 4J1 Canada

Print management and distribution
Print Konsult
187, 401-9th Avenue SW, Calgary, AB, T2P 3C5 Canada

Canadian Cataloguing in Publication Data

Premkumar, Kalyani, 1959-
  Pathology A to Z

  Includes bibliographical references and index.
  ISBN 0-9680730-0-X

  1. Pathology—Handbooks, manuals, etc. 2. Massage therapy-
-Handbooks, manuals etc. I. Title.
  RB118.P73 1996   616.07   C96-910582-7

Produced in Canada

Preface

*T*here has been a tremendous change in health care systems in the recent past around the world, particularly in North America. Emphasis is being placed on holistic care, especially by the public. Alternative forms of therapy such as massage, acupuncture, acupressure and reflexology among others are gaining respect and acceptance. It is a time for recruiting new members into the health care team which until now comprised primarily of Medical Practitioners. The time is ripe for alternative health professionals to claim their place in the health care team.

Undoubtedly, to become fully accepted members of the health care team, it is vital for Holistic Health Practitioners to equip themselves with the knowledge about diseases and their causes that has been painstakingly accumulated over years of scientific research. It is also important to understand and be fluent with the language of medicine, in order to communicate effectively with other members of the team. This is the first step that has to be taken to bridge the gap that exists between Medical and Alternative Health Practitioners. Several measures are being taken to help this process especially in the field of Massage Therapy. For instance, the curriculum in Massage Therapy Colleges is being scrutinized in many provinces of Canada, and more stringent licensing procedures are being introduced.

While these changes are taking place, there is a growing realization that there is a lack of printed resources that cater specifically to the needs of Massage Therapists. At present, both students and practitioners are forced to wade through voluminous literature of medicine to discover simple but important details relevant to their practice. What is the cause of a disease they encounter? Is it infectious? Can the client be harmed by massage? Can the Therapist be harmed by contact with the client? What are the precautions that should be taken? are few of the questions that arise constantly in a Massage Therapist's mind. Realizing this urgent need, this handbook of Pathology has been written to serve as a ready reckoner for Massage Therapists and other Holistic Health Practitioners.

Acknowledgments

This book could not have been written without the support of my husband and teammate, Prem, who believed in my capabilities, encouraged and urged (drove) me on to completion.

The enthusiasm and patience of my loving children, Vivian and Kamini, who endured the long hours I spent away from them during the preparation of this book made it possible.

The insight to the book industry provided by the Publishers and the professionalism of the Print Managers certainly made this maiden venture happen.

The contribution of the color slides by Dr. Tom Enta is gratefully acknowledged.

- Kalyani Premkumar

Contents

Foreword

*T*he practice of massage has changed dramatically over the past few years in North America. Massage, which was once regarded as a hobby practiced by "flaky" individuals, is now recognized as a valid health care modality provided by highly trained therapists. The public's demand for massage therapy as a tool to deal with stress, pain and various pathological conditions is based on an increasing awareness of its incredible effectiveness in helping the body heal itself when administered under the proper conditions.

A solid understanding of how the body works, becomes unwell and heals itself is what distinguishes a person as a therapist rather than a hobbyist. With this knowledge, the therapist is able to hone in on which specific massage techniques to apply and where, thus maximizing the potential for the healing process to take place. This understanding comes from training and experience.

Both students and practicing massage therapists will welcome Dr. Premkumar's "Pathology A to Z - a Handbook for Massage Therapists". It will help them reach a high level of understanding of the relationship between massage and pathological conditions. It is not intended as a textbook that explains what this relationship is and how it works, but rather as a study guide or quick reference to enrich or refresh the memory of what the condition is and what relevance massage therapy has to it. In the massage therapy field, we have been waiting for such a reference for a long time.

There are few people as qualified as Dr. Premkumar to produce this type of reference guide. She has the medical training to give her the expertise to explain pathologies, as well as the massage therapy training which enables her to make the relevant connections for massage therapists to understand those pathologies and provide appropriate treatments.

In addition, Dr. Premkumar is an adult educator who knows how to present material in a user-friendly fashion. The alphabetized format of the pathological conditions is ideal for quick reference. The information under each condition and in the other two sections on common drugs and control of infections is concise, accurate (to today's understanding) and relevant to the massage therapist. Dr. Premkumar recognizes that much of what is known about the use and effectiveness of therapeutic massage is based on empirical data; therefore, she has provided space for the owner of the book to add personal notes based on experience directly after each pathology.

"Pathology A to Z - A Handbook for Massage Therapists" is a must-have resource that every massage therapy student and practicing massage therapist will find very useful.

Sylvia Muiznieks, B.Sc., R.M.T.
Program Administrator, Massage Therapy Training Institute
Mount Royal College, Calgary, Alberta, Canada

Foreword

*L*ike all professions, medicine has its own unique vocabulary - its own terms, its own shorthand, special acronyms and definitions. A good medical dictionary is one of the first books which the beginning student must have. As the students' learning progresses a personal library that covers many different disciplines grows to constitute a body of knowledge that is used for their practice of medicine.

Pathology is an important part of medicine which has traditionally concentrated on the changes in the structure of cells, tissues and organs resulting from a myriad of different disease processes. Accordingly, a pathologist can diagnose a cancer from minute tissue samples (biopsies) by looking at the cellular changes, or can conduct a post mortem to ascertain the cause of an untimely death. The disease process itself alters cellular and organ function ultimately affecting the health and well-being of the patient. It is this study of the biology of disease that helps one understand the changing signs and symptoms as the severity and stage of the disease progress. In this way, pathology has given us a better foundation for understanding the natural evolution of a disease, which in turn leads to more rational and sounder clinical practice.

In this book, Dr. Premkumar presents a series of standardized descriptions of different diseases with respect to their causes, signs and symptoms, and risk factors. In this way she emphasizes the relevance of pathology to clinical medicine. At the same time, one should never forget that there are many clinical dysfunctions and symptomatologies that cannot be correlated to an obvious cellular or tissue abnormality. This is especially true in the entire area of psychosomatic medicine.

Frequently a referral letter may mention or clients will tell the therapist that they suffer from a specific disease. This book gives massage therapists enough information to understand the basic problems associated with many different diseases and any specific implications they may have for therapy. Under the section, Caution and Recommendations to Therapists, Dr. Premkumar includes a warning if the disease is contagious and special precautions need to be taken.

I have no doubt that this book will serve a valuable function as a quick reference for students and practitioners of massage therapy. It should find an important place in every practitioners' library. At the same time it should also appeal to many other allied health professionals.

John S. Baumber, Ph.D., M.D.,
Professor,
Department of Physiology and Biophysics
& Office of Medical Education
Faculty of Medicine, University of Calgary, Calgary, Alberta, Canada

Introduction to the book

*T*he book has been organized alphabetically, according to diseases. As well, it has disease-wise and body-system wise indices, to assist the reader in locating diseases with more than one name. Every disease has been dealt with using a uniform format for better readability and quick reference.

Each disease has a short description followed by the Cause, Signs and Symptoms, Risk factors and Caution and Recommendations to Therapists. The primary body system affected by the disease has also been indicated. Space has been allocated under each disease for recording individual observations and notes. This space can also be utilized for noting other forms of treatment for that particular disorder - such as Aromatherapy, Acupressure etc., that the Holistic Practitioner is familiar with. Color plates have been included to illustrate some of the common skin ailments. Also, Figures have been inserted wherever appropriate beside the description of the condition.

The Glossary provided for medical terms used in the book will be helpful to understand unfamiliar terminology. The side effects of some of the common drugs is an additional feature to alert Therapists while treating clients under medical management. Addresses of relevant resources and associations in Canada and United States, have been added to enable Practitioners access recent advances made, locate local support groups and for client education. A separate section on Strategies for prevention of infection and safe practice, gives simple precautions that can be adapted to combat infectious diseases.

The objective of this book is to help the reader understand more about diseases that have been **diagnosed by a Physician**, and to serve as a guideline, so that the client can be urged to a state of total well-being using non-invasive and alternative forms of therapy. It is envisaged that this book will help Holistic Practitioners broaden their outlook and attitude to make them feel comfortable as an accepted member of the health care team.

IT IS EMPHASIZED THAT THIS IS NOT A MEDICAL MANUAL TO HELP HOLISTIC PRACTITIONERS DIAGNOSE AND TREAT DISEASES, AND IT MAY NOT BE USED FOR SUCH PURPOSES.

- Author

Abortion (Miscarriage)

The spontaneous or induced expulsion of the products of conception from the uterus before 20 weeks of pregnancy.

Cause:

Spontaneous abortion could be due to many reasons. Abnormal development of the embryo due to genetic defects, faults in the implantation of the embryo, abnormal positioning of the placenta are some of the causes. Maternal factors such as infection, severe malnutrition, abnormal reproductive organs such as incompetent cervix, injury, hormonal imbalances and blood group incompatibility may also produce spontaneous abortions.

Signs and Symptoms:

Abortions may be preceded by a pink or brown discharge from the vagina before the onset of cramps, severe bleeding and expulsion of the contents of the uterus. If all the products are not expelled, the cramps and bleeding continue for days.

Risk factors:

See Cause.

Caution and Recommendations to Therapists:

In general, do not massage the lower abdomen in the early stages of pregnancy. If a client is prone to spontaneous abortions and is pregnant, always consult the Obstetrician before massaging. Pregnancy massage with the client seated, lying on the side or any other comfortable position, can be done if cleared by the Obstetrician. In any case, the massage should be gentle and relaxing, and for a shorter duration. Fascial techniques to the low back should be avoided as also the use of potent essential oils. Lavender (for its calming effect), neroli (for its relaxing effects on smooth muscles of the gut), tangerine (for its uplifting effect) in a 1% dilution, have been recommended by some for use during pregnancy.

Notes:

Sponatneous abortions are of many types. *Threatened abortion* is the condition when there is slight bleeding from the vagina. About 50% of such pregnancies are not aborted. *Inevitable abortion* is when the cervix dilates and abortion is definite. When parts of the products are retained in the uterus, it is termed as *incomplete abortion*. *Complete abortion* indicates complete expulsion of the products with minimal bleeding. *Missed abortion* is when the fetus is retained in the uterus for two months or more even after its death.

A person is said to have *habitual abortion* when there is spontaneous loss of three or more pregnancies. When there is infection associated with abortion, it is termed *septic abortion.*

Acne Conglobata

A chronic inflammatory skin disorder affecting the sebaceous glands and hair follicles.

Cause:

Irritation produced by components of sebum from the sebaceous glands escaping into the dermis is responsible for the inflammation. The cause of acne is unknown and many factors influence its course (see risk factors).

Signs and Symptoms:

Blackheads, pustules, abscesses, nodules and cysts can be seen in any area of the trunk, face and thighs. The secretions from the lesions may be foul smelling, watery or pustular. Scars may be seen from previous lesions.

Risk factors:

It is common in middle age. It is more common in men than women. High fat diet, food products such as chocolate, makeup, infection by Propionibacterium acnes organism, stress, increased activity and proliferation of sebum producing cells are all predisposing factors.

Caution and Recommendations to Therapists:

Acne is not contagious, neither can it be spread from one region of the body to another by touch. Avoid massaging the affected area if there is extensive inflammation. Some clients may like light massage of the face without oil, so judgment on an individual basis should be made. Wash hands thoroughly before massaging the face in such clients as super infection can be introduced by unclean, oily hands. Many clients with acne are self-conscious, with low self-esteem because of its appearance. Therapists need to treat such clients with special care.

Clients may be on oral steroid therapy for the condition and the overall immunity may be lowered as a result. The therapists should not treat such clients if harboring any kind of infection, as it may spread to the client.

Notes: ⎯⎯⎯⎯⎯⎯⎯⎯⎯⎯⎯⎯⎯⎯⎯⎯⎯⎯⎯⎯⎯⎯⎯⎯⎯⎯⎯

Acne Rosacea

A chronic inflammatory skin disorder affecting the sebaceous glands and hair follicles.

Cause:

See Acne Conglobata.

Signs and Symptoms:

It begins slowly as redness with or without blackheads, pustules, abscesses, nodules and cysts, over the nose, cheeks, chin and forehead. In chronic cases, it may result in irregular, thickening of the skin over the nose.

Risk factors:

It is common in middle aged and elderly adults. Heat, cold, sunlight, hot liquids, highly seasoned foods, alcohol, high fat diet, food products such as chocolate, makeup, infection by Propionibacterium acnes organism, stress, factors producing increased activity and proliferation of sebum producing cells are all risk factors.

Caution and Recommendations to Therapists:

See Acne Conglobata. Avoid hot or cold packs as it may worsen the condition.

Notes: ⎯⎯⎯⎯⎯⎯⎯⎯⎯⎯⎯⎯⎯⎯⎯⎯⎯⎯⎯⎯⎯⎯⎯⎯⎯⎯⎯

Acne Vulgaris

An inflammatory skin disorder affecting the sebaceous glands and hair follicles.

Cause:

See Acne Conglobata.

Signs and Symptoms:

There is formation of blackheads, papules and pustules and inflammation in the face, and neck. It may also be seen in the back, shoulders and chest. (see Appendix I figure 1)

Risk factors:

See Acne Conglobata.

Caution and Recommendations to Therapists:

See Acne Conglobata.

Notes

Acquired Immunodeficiency Syndrome
(AIDS, Human Immunodeficiency Virus infection)

Lymphatic, Cardiovascular, Pulmonary, Nervous systems

A viral infection that progressively destroys the immunity of the individual.

Cause:

It is caused by the RNA virus - Human Immunodeficiency Virus Type I/ Type II (HIV). The virus primarily affects the T lymphocytes which are responsible for cell-mediated immunity (the type of immunity that comes into play in skin graft rejection etc.). However, it does affect other forms of immunity too. AIDS victims become vulnerable to infections that do not affect normal individuals. Also, infections that produce only mild symptoms otherwise, may produce severe symptoms in them. They are also prone to unusual cancers.

It is transmitted by contact with infected blood or body fluids. Intercourse, (anal/vaginal), transfusion of contaminated blood or blood products, sharing of contaminated needles, transmission to the fetus from infected mothers through the placenta are some of the routes through which the virus is transmitted. There is growing evidence that it is not transmitted by casual social or household contact.

On an average, the time between exposure to the virus and diagnosis is 8-10 years. But the incubation period may be shorter or longer. Initially, the presence of the virus is detected only by laboratory tests. Later, symptoms due to the deficient immune state is seen. There is a wide variation in the way the disease presents and the time between acute infection and onset of symptoms.

Signs and Symptoms:

The signs and symptoms are variable. Initially, the person may exhibit only flu-like symptoms and remain asymptomatic for many years. Later, the infection process may present as opportunistic infections (infections that do not affect normal individuals) and unusual cancers. Some of the common infections and cancers that are seen in AIDS infection are fungal infections, Tuberculosis, Herpes virus infection, pneumonia, sarcomas and lymphomas. In some, it presents as autoimmunity where the body's immune cells attack self eg. as arthritis, or as neurological problems - encephalitis, dementia or peripheral neuritis. There may be generalized enlargement of lymph nodes, weight loss, fatigue, night sweats and fever.

Risk factors:

Homosexual and bisexual individuals, intravenous drug users, those requiring recurrent transfusions of blood or blood products and heterosexual partners of the above groups are all at risk. There is a high incidence of AIDS in infants born to infected mothers.

Caution and Recommendations to Therapists:

The HIV epidemic has challenged the thinking about fundamental ethical and legal issues such as confidentiality, right to privacy, informed consent etc. It has challenged the codes that require health professionals such as nurses and doctors to provide service to all people without regard for socioeconomic status or nature of health problems.

Although it is unlikely for Massage Therapists to come in contact with blood or body fluids of clients, in general, special precautions have to be taken. It is advisable for Massage Therapists to wear gloves, or refrain from treating any client if the Therapist has an open wound. The treatment regime has to be individualized as AIDS presents in very many ways. A full body relaxation massage of short duration is recommended. Since the disease affects the immunity of the individual, it should be ensured that the client is not exposed to any form of infection in the clinic. AIDS clients may have diseases like tuberculosis, herpes, hepatitis B, among others. Special precautions have to be taken to prevent spread of such diseases to the Therapist.

It is possible for the Therapist to transmit negative feelings to the client through touch. If the Therapist is uncomfortable massaging an individual diagnosed to have AIDS, it may be better to refer the client to another Therapist who is comfortable, rather than force oneself to give an ineffective massage.

If there has been an exposure to blood or body fluids inadvertently, immediately, scrub the site vigorously with a disinfectant solution such as 10% povidone iodine and wash under running water for 10 minutes (this *may* help remove the HIV cells from site). Report immediately to a Medical Service.

Many support groups are available for those affected by AIDS. Refer client to a local support group (see Appendix IV).

Notes: _____

One of the tests performed to indicate exposure to AIDS is the Enzyme-linked immunosorbent assay test (ELISA). This identifies the presence of antibodies to the AIDS virus. If this is positive more sophisticated tests are performed. However, testing for antibodies alone is not reliable as it may take from a few weeks to many months for antibody production to reach detectable levels.

Adhesive Capsulitis (Frozen shoulder, Scapulocostal syndrome, Calcific tendinitis of the rotator cuff, Subacromial fibrosis, Pericapsulitis, Acromioclavicular arthritis)

Musculoskeletal system

A disorder of the shoulder joint caused by tightening of the joint capsule.

Cause:

The cause is not known in most situations. It may be caused by misalignment of the scapula with the humerus as in individuals with kyphosis. It may also be due to the spread of inflammation from lesions of the rotator cuff with resultant fibrosis of the capsule. Rarely, degenerative shoulder joint disease, rheumatoid arthritis, and prolonged immobilization can cause this condition.

Signs and Symptoms:

There is a slow restriction of movement of the arm to the point of affecting daily activities such as combing hair. It may be associated with gradual onset of a dull ache. The client finds it difficult to abduct and flex the arm and has difficulty moving the arm to the back. There is limitation of external rotation, abduction, flexion and internal rotation of shoulder. There is pain referred to the C5,C6 area. In acute frozen shoulder, the pain may radiate to below the elbow. Nocturnal pain is common. In chronic conditions, nocturnal pain is absent and pain is felt only on stretching the capsule.

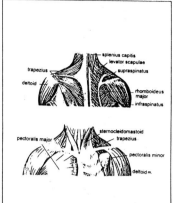

Risk factors:

This condition is more common in women.

Caution and Recommendations to Therapists:

In acute frozen shoulder, ice or superficial heat reduce pain and muscle guarding. The aim is to maintain and slowly increase the range of movement. Use capsular stretching procedures with the clients arm hanging over the side of the table. In the chronic stage, the aim is to stretch the capsule - especially the antero-inferior area. Muscle spasms of the back should also be addressed. Specifically, the muscles around the shoulder girdle, pectoralis major and minor, and rotator cuff muscles should be focussed upon. The biceps, triceps, subscapularis and deltoid should be thoroughly massaged. Improvement occurs very slowly and awareness of this reduces frustration in the part of the massage therapist and the client.

Work in close conjunction with a physiotherapist. Encourage client to do stretching and strengthening exercises to improve the range of motion and strength of muscles. Some of the effective exercises include standing beside a wall and walking the fingers up the wall as high as possible. This helps with abduction of the shoulder. Another effective exercise is the pendulum swing where the client leans forward waist down while holding onto a support about a foot away from the body, while the affected arm hangs loose. The arm is then slowly moved in circles of different diameters.

Schedules lasting for half an hour, three times a week for three weeks followed by twice a week for two weeks, and modified thereafter according to improvement is the recommended regimen.

Notes: _____

It is treated surgically or by injection of steroids into the joint capsule.

Adrenogenital syndrome

It includes a spectrum of disorders resulting from abnormality in the synthesis of adrenocortical hormones.

Cause:

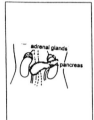

It is usually caused by a lack of specific enzymes required for the synthesis of the steroidal hormones in the adrenal cortex. It is transmitted to a child from a parent with the defective gene (congenital adrenal hyperplasia). Since many enzymes are required for synthesis and the synthesis is in the form of a cascade, lack of one enzyme results in accumulation of the precursors. Thus there is an excess of androgens (hormones that are responsible for development of the reproductive organs). Aldosterone (hormone regulating sodium and water levels in the body), and corticosteroids (hormone regulating metabolism of fat, carbohydrate and protein) levels are also low.

Signs and Symptoms:

The symptoms vary according to the sex and age. In new born females, the external genitalia is abnormal. The clitoris is enlarged and resembles a penis, and the labia majora are fused to each other. In newborn males, there is no obvious abnormality. At puberty, females do not start menstrual periods. There is deepening of voice and growth of facial hair. The skin is oily and acne is common. The loss of fluid and sodium produces signs of dehydration. The condition is difficult to diagnose in males.

Risk factors:

It is more common in females than males.

Caution and Recommendations to Therapists:

Encourage client to take the prescribed replacement hormonal therapy regularly.

Notes:

The cause is identified and treated accordingly. The deficient hormones are replaced by daily administration.

Adult Respiratory Distress Syndrome
(ARDS, Shock lung)

Difficulty in breathing brought on by stiffening of the lung by fluid accumulation.

Cause:

The lung capillaries become more leaky allowing fluid to get into the spaces between the cells and thereby stiffen the lung. This leads to difficulty in inflating the lung and reduced exchange of oxygen.

Signs and Symptoms:

It presents as difficulty in breathing, noisy and rapid, labored respiration. It progresses to restlessness, mental disorientation and if left uncorrected to heart failure and death.

Risk factors:

Entry of stomach contents into the respiratory tract, trauma, pneumonia, smoke or chemical inhalation that produce inflammation and drowning are risk factors. Rarely, it may be a complication of tuberculosis.

Caution and Recommendations to Therapists:

The condition has to be treated in hospital under close monitoring of respiratory rate and other vital signs. Massage can help maintain joint mobility and range of motion of various joints while the individual is confined to bed. A gentle relaxation massage can help reduce stress in these highly stressed individuals. More time should be spent on massaging the accessory muscles of respiration including the sternocleidomastoid, pectoralis, latissimus dorsi and neck muscles.

Notes: ————————————————————————————————

Alzheimer's disease (Primary degenerative dementia)

A progressive form of mental disorder that results in deterioration of the intellect (dementia), severe enough to affect the performance of the person socially and in their occupation.

Cause:

The cause is unknown, but various factors have been implicated. It could be due to deficiencies of certain neurotransmitters such as acetylcholine, norepinephrine and somatostatin. Viral factors, hereditary, immunological and environmental factors have also been implicated. There is slow loss and atrophy of brain tissue particularly in the temporal and frontal lobe. There is accumulation of a protein (beta amyloid precursor protein) in and around neurons and blood vessels of the brain that interfere with the transmission of nerve impulses.

Signs and Symptoms:

It starts very slowly with forgetfulness, learning difficulties, difficulty in concentrating and lack of personal hygiene. It then progresses to language, communication difficulties and lack of motor coordination. It is accompanied by personality changes. Finally, the individual has urinary and fecal incontinence and is unable to recognize family and friends. Siezures may also occur. The person also becomes more susceptible to infection.

Risk factors:

There may be a family history of the disease. It occurs in middle and late life. It is more common in people with Down's syndrome. Increased intake of aluminium - as in cooking in aluminium utensils, excessive use of aluminium containing antacids have also been implicated as risk factors.

Caution and Recommendations to Therapists:

Alzhiemer's disease is not infectious. A full body relaxation massage helps to soothe the individuals. Vary the duration of massage according to individual tolerance. As the disease progresses the motor function deteriorates. The aim should be to prevent joint stiffening and contractures and to maintain mobility. Passively move all joints. Use transverse friction around joints. Do not overstimulate hypertonic muscles. Massage to antagonist muscles can help relax affected muscles. Since these individuals are bedridden in late stages, watch for bed sores. Avoid massaging over a wide area around bed sores. Research has shown that massaging over and around bed sores worsen the condition and causes more damage to tissues. Since these individuals are more susceptible to infection do not massage when you have even a mild infection. Encourage client to exercise. Keep addresses of local support groups handy. (Refer to Appendix IV).

Notes: _____

There is no known cure yet. Drugs are given to increase the levels of neurotransmitters and increase blood flow and thereby oxygen to the brain.

Amputation

Musculoskeletal, Nervous systems

Removal of part of a limb when its survival compromises the health or life of the client.

Cause:

Amputations are done when the blood supply to parts of the body are severely compromised leading to gangrene formation or infection. The cause of pain symptoms such as Phantom Limb pain in amputees cannot be fully explained by a single mechanism. It has been attributed to changes in the peripheral, autonomic and central nervous system after amputation.

Signs and Symptoms:

Clients after amputation often have Phantom Limb pain. Phantom limb has been described as having a tingling feeling or a feeling of a definite shape of the amputated limb. The shape may take the form of the real limb initially, but later change in shape. Cramping, shooting, crushing or burning pain may be felt in this area, starting immediately, or days or months later. Later other zones may become sensitized and act as triggers for phantom pain. The pain may also be aggravated by emotions, stress, urination or defecation.

Risk Factors:

Amputation may be done on clients with a) arteriosclerosis where the diminished blood supply has resulted in gangrene; b) severe trauma to the limb; c) malignant tumors; and d) complications of diabetes leading to gangrene.

Caution and Recommendations to Therapists:

Since the pain mechanism changes with time, the therapeutic approach also has to be modified according to individual needs. Obtain a detailed history of triggers that produce Phantom limb pain. Even gentle touch, warmth and other painless stimuli in an area away from the amputation site can be triggers. Application of ice, or quick light percussion strokes of the amputated limb and stump may help relieve phantom pain.

Massage is given after the stumps have healed completely. Use passive movements to loosen the stiffened joints in the area. Effleurage is used to reduce edema and increase the circulation. Massage muscles of the shoulders, back, arms and trunk to reduce fatigue and pain in muscles that are used for working with crutches or prosthesis.

Notes:

Phantom limb has been treated with anaesthetic blockage of trigger sites, or by excessive stimulation. Vigorous vibration of the stump have also been used successfully. Other modes of treatment have been placement of electrodes in the dorsal column of the spinal cord.

Amyotrophic Lateral Sclerosis (ALS, Lou Gehrig's disease)

Nervous system

A progressive disease of the motor neurons that produces atrophy of muscles.

Cause:

The cause is unknown. It has been found to be hereditary in a few cases where the onset of the disease has been in childhood or early adulthood. The disease produces death of the lower motor neuron (neurons from the brain and spinal cord that go directly to the muscle) as well as upper motor neurons (neurons from the brain that modify the actions of lower motor neurons). The sensory neurons, the autonomic regulation, control of movement and the intellect are intact.

Signs and Symptoms:

Due to the death of the upper motor neurons, the person has increased tone of muscles, exaggerated reflexes, weakness, and lack of fine control over movements. The affectation of the lower motor neuron results in flaccidity (lack of tone), atrophy and weakness of muscles. Typically this disease begins with weakness and atrophy of the small muscles of the hand. It progresses to affect other limbs, neck and face. In severe cases the muscles of the pharynx, palate, tongue and other regions are affected producing difficulty in speech and swallowing. Affectation of the respiratory muscles can result in labored breathing and death.

Risk factors:

It usually begins between the ages of 40-70. It affects men more than women. In the early onset disease which is hereditary, both men and women are affected equally.

Caution and Recommendations to Therapists:

Take time to assess the client thoroughly. Since both upper and lower motor neurons can be affected, the tone may be increased in some groups of muscles while others are flaccid with marked atrophy. Contractures may also be present. Remember that the intellect as well as the sensory system is intact. This is one disease which will pose a tremendous challenge to the massage therapist as the treatment options have to be varied since the presentation changes from day to day. The aim is to reduce tone in regions with increased tone - so a relaxation massage is required here with increased use of strokes like effleurage and gentle friction. In regions with decreased tone a stimulatory massage is required with more use of pertrissage. Use friction strokes to prevent adhesions. Perform passive range of motion movements of all joints to prevent joint stiffness. Massage has been shown to increase circulation in muscles. This may help alleviate the muscle cramps that these clients often get. Encourage clients to join support groups in the local area. Refer to Appendix IV for resources.

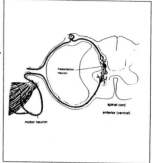

Notes: _____

There is no treatment as yet that can stop the progress of the disease. Only supportive treatment is available. The average survival time is 2-5 years.

Anemia
Cardiovascular system

A condition where the hemoglobin level in the blood is below normal.

Cause:

Anemia may be due to various causes. A reduced number of red blood cells can result in anemia. Conditions that destroy the bone marrow such as tumors and exposure to radiation can result in aplastic anemia. Here the production of platelets and white blood cells are affected in addition to red blood cells.

Conditions that lead to excessive blood loss can also cause anemia. The blood loss could be acute as after injuries, vomiting of blood (esophageal varices rupture), coughing of blood (can occur in Tuberculosis), blood loss in the feces (hemorrhoids, colon tumors, peptic ulcers, ulcerative colitis, worm infestation etc.) or profuse menstruation in women (endometriosis, fibroids etc.). Bleeding disorders like hemophilia where there is a lack of clotting factors can result in excessive blood loss and anemia.

Anemia may also result if the components for manufacture of hemoglobin are inadequate. Protein, iron, vitamin B12 or folic acid deficiency can lead to this type of anemia. Protein deficiency can be seen in malabsorption syndrome or malnutrition. Iron deficiency can occur due to reduced intake or increased need as during pregnancy. Deficiency of vitamin B12 or folic acid can follow reduced intake or lack of intrinsic factor in the stomach. The intrinsic factor secreted in the stomach is required for proper absorption of vitamin B12 in the ileum. This type of anemia is called pernicious anemia. Increased destruction of red cells can also lead to anemia. This occurs when the spleen is overactive, or if the red cells are abnormal. In certain genetic disorders like thalassemia and sickle cell anemia, the structure of the hemoglobin is abnormal and the red cells are destroyed prematurely.

Signs and Symptoms:

Initially, there are no specific symptoms. The person fatigues easily, is listless, irritable and is unable to concentrate. There is also a greater susceptibility to infections. Pallor may be seen. The nails tend to become brittle and spoon shaped. Cracking of the corners of the mouth and smoothness of tongue are other symptoms. In severe cases, there may be numbness and tingling of the fingers. Other associated symptoms and signs are seen depending on the type of anemia.

Risk factors:

See Cause.

Caution and Recommendations to Therapists:

Advice clients who appear abnormally pale to see a physician and get their hemoglobin levels checked.

If the anemia is due to bleeding disorders, care should be taken not to use excessive pressure as they tend to bruise easily and bleeding can occur under the skin. It should also be remembered that anemic individuals are susceptible to infections. It should be ensured that they are not exposed to any infection in the clinic. Refer to Appendix IV for resources,

Notes: _____

It is important to identify the cause of anemia before treating it. Nutritional deficiency anemias can be prevented by the intake of a well balanced diet that includes, red meats, green vegetables, eggs, whole wheat, milk etc. Iron supplements are required when the needs are increased as during pregnancy and in nursing mothers.

Aneurysm

An abnormal localized dilatation of an artery.

Cause:

Any condition which causes weakening of the arterial wall can lead to an aneurysm. Dissecting aneurysms - the type which results in hemorrhage into the vessel wall are common in clients with hypertension and those with connective tissue disorders (eg. Marfan's syndrome).

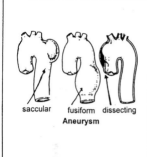

saccular   fusiform   dissecting
Aneurysm

Signs and Symptoms:

Often, aneurysms are asymptomatic and may only be diagnosed on rupturing. With aneurysms of the thoracic aorta, the client may have pain in the back, neck, or behind the sternum. Difficulty in breathing, dry cough or noisy breathing, hoarseness of voice may be present due to the pressure of the dilated vessel on the surrounding tissue.

Pressure on the superior vena cava may result in edema of the face and neck and engorgement of neck veins. Sometimes, the client may present with a pulsating mass.

Aneurysm can occur in any artery. Rupture of an aneurysm in an artery in the brain can be a cause of sudden death.

Risk factors:

Congenital defects, trauma, infections, arteriosclerosis, hypertension and connective tissue disorders predispose to this condition.

Caution and Recommendations to Therapists:

Consult physician before embarking on deep abdominal massage, on clients with history of hypertension or atherosclerosis. Heavy abdominal massage in clients with abdominal aortic aneurysm can result in rupture, extensive bleeding and death. Avoid massage over any mass that is pulsating.

Notes:

Angina Pectoris (Ischemic Heart Disease)

(Latin - to choke)   Cardiovascular system

It is a form of heart disease produced by inadequate blood supply to the walls of the heart.

Cause:

The classical type of angina is associated with narrowing of the coronary arteries by atherosclerosis. The symptoms are usually precipitated by exercise. The variant type of angina is brought on by spasm of the coronaries and can occur at rest or at night.

Signs and Symptoms:

The disease presents as recurring pain lasting for a short duration. The pain or pressure sensation may be felt over the chest or posterior to the sternum and may radiate to the shoulder, arm, jaw, or other areas of the chest. The pain is usually described as constricting, squeezing or suffocating. In the classical types, the symptoms are precipitated by exercise. In the variant type, the pain can occur at rest or at night. In the unstable type the pain becomes progressively severe, lasting longer. This type can lead to myocardial infarction.

Risk factors:

Family history of angina, hypertension, obesity, smoking, diabetes mellitus, stress, sedentary life-style and high cholesterol levels in the blood are all risk factors.

Caution and Recommendations to Therapists:

Massage can help these clients by reducing stress levels. Stress predisposes to an anginal attack. Massage also reduces the activity of the sympathetic nervous system which is partly responsible for coronary vasoconstriction. Sudden exposure to extreme cold or heat can bring on an attack. So keep the client warm, and avoid extreme fluctuations in temperature when using heat or cold packs. If a client has an attack on the table, bring him/her up to a sitting or standing position as this reduces the load on the heart and call for help. Always make sure that a client diagnosed to have angina has the prescription drugs handy, while coming for massage. Keep the telephone number of the client's physician in your records.

Notes: ——————— ——————————————————————————————

Ankylosing spondylitis
(Spondylitis, Ankylopoietica)

Musculoskeletal system

An inflammatory disease of the axial skeleton.

Cause:

The cause is unknown. The presence of large macrophages in the acute stages suggest an immune response.

Signs and Symptoms:

It affects the sacro-iliac joints, intervertebral disk spaces and costo-vertebral joints commonly. Rarely, it affects the large synovial joints like hips, knees and shoulders. Fibrosis, calcification, ossification and stiffening of the joints are seen. The spine becomes rigid and bamboo like. The disease has exacerbations and remissions.

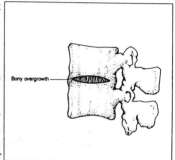

Typically, the client complains of persistent or intermittent low back pain. The pain becomes worse at rest and is reduced by mild activity. The pain may also radiate to the thigh. There is loss of mobility of the vertebral column and the curvature of the lumbar region is slowly lost. In late stages the spine gets fixed. If the costovertebral joints are fixed it can affect the lung volume. Kyphosis is present when the thoracic or cervical regions are affected and the weight of the head compresses the vertebral bodies and bends the spine forward. The head is therefore hyper-extended to help maintain the field of vision.

Ankylosing spondylitis may be accompanied by weight loss, fever and fatigue. Osteoporosis may also be present. Complications include fractures, subluxation of the spine and spinal cord compression.

Risk factors:

It is more common in North America. The disease is more severe in men. It occurs at any age but the incidence is higher in the 20-30 age group.

Caution and Recommendations to Therapists:

The client should be positioned according to individual comfort. In clients with kyphosis extra cushioning in the neck region may be needed.

The aim is to retain the mobility of the joints, to strengthen weak muscles and to stretch tight ones. Do not try to forcibly mobilize ankylosed joints. Gentle massage should be given to the back and limbs. Hot packs are very helpful to ease the pain.

Advice clients to sleep in a supine position if possible. Encourage client to do breathing exercises regularly to mobilize the thorax.

Notes: ───

Anterior compartment syndrome

Musculoskeletal system

A collection of signs and symptoms produced by increased pressure and consequent reduced blood flow to a closed muscle compartment in the leg.

Cause:

In the leg a compact compartment is formed between the tibia and fibula and an unyielding fascia around the muscles in the anterior compartment. The muscles tibialis anterior, extensor hallucis longus, extensor digitorum longus, peroneus tertius, the peroneal nerve and blood vessels lie in this compartment. Any condition that increases the pressure in the compartment compromises the blood supply to the soft tissue resulting in the characteristic symptoms.

Signs and Symptoms:

There is a tight feeling in the calf region with pain, tenderness, numbness and tingling. The symptoms develop slowly but progress steadily and are pronounced on using the leg. Like angina pectoris, the pain begins after using the limb to the same extent every time. The pain may be produced even on stretching the muscle.

Risk factors:

It is usually caused by overuse and repetitive stress to the muscles in this compartment. The stress results in inflammation and swelling of the tissue in this confined space.

Caution and Recommendations to Therapists:

The limb should be positioned in level with the heart. Elevation may reduce the blood flow to the already compromised tissue. Placing the limb in a dependent position may increase the venous congestion due to the effect of gravity. In the acute stage, measures to reduce the inflammation and swelling are helpful. Rest and ice application have been found to be beneficial. The thighs should be massaged well, using broad strokes like effleurage and petrissage to increase venous and lymphatic drainage.

In the subacute stage, heat can be applied to soften the connective tissue. Suitable strokes such as cross fibre friction are used to stretch the tight fascia followed by ice application. However, Such techniques should be avoided if it is too painful. In those with lowered sensation, care should be taken not to use excessive pressure as the feedback from the client is likely to be inadequate.

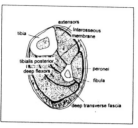

Notes: _____

The condition is diagnosed by measuring the pressure in the compartment . If the symptoms are chronic or severe, surgery may be done to reduce the pressure.

Appendicitis
Gastrointestinal system

The inflammation of the vermiform appendix.

Cause:

The inflammation is a result of obstruction to the lumen of the appendix by faeces, or due to twisting. The appendix becomes swollen and red, and if the obstruction persists death of tissue occurs with perforation of the appendix and spilling of the contents into the abdominal cavity producing toxic reactions.

Signs and Symptoms:

Sites of referred pain

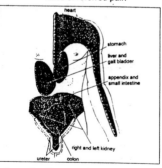

The person experiences a vague pain below the sternum and around the umbilicus. The location of the pain is different from the actual position of the appendix as the pain is referred to this area. The pain intensifies over a few hours and becomes colicky (spasmodic) in nature. When the inflammation spreads to the peritoneal covering, the pain is localized to the right lower quadrant of the abdomen. The abdominal muscles over the area go into spasm and become boardlike. The person walks bent over, or lies with the right hip flexed to reduce the pain. Fever, nausea and vomiting accompany the pain. Immediate surgery is required if complications of abscess formation, peritonitis or spread of infection to other areas are to be combated.

Risk factors:

It can occur at any age but is frequent between 5-30 years of age.

Caution and Recommendations to Therapists:

Do not massage the abdomen if a person complains of pain resembling that of appendicitis as massage can rupture the inflamed appendix. Refer to a physician immediately.

Notes: _____

Appendix is a wormlike structure of 3-6 inches in length, that is attached to the cecum. The pain produced by appendicitis can resemble that of many other conditions like gastritis, renal stones, pancreatitis, ovarian cyst, diseases of the uterus and inflammation of other areas of the bowel.

Arthritis - gouty (Gout)   Muslculoskeletal system

A joint disorder due to deposition of crystals.

Cause:

Gout is caused by deposition of monosodium urate or uric acid crystals in the joint cavity. The crystals attract leucocytes which in turn release lysosomal enzymes that trigger inflammation. The deposition of crystals in joints is due to the higher levels of urate in the serum either due to decreased elimination or increased production.

Signs and Symptoms:

There is an acute onset of pain, redness and swelling of the joint. It affects the peripheral joints-commonly the metatarsophalangeal joint of the big toe.

Risk factors:

Primary gout is more common in men between the ages of 40 and 60. In women, those who are postmenopausal are affected. It has been associated with genetic defects in the metabolism of purine.The attack of gout may be precipitated by certain drugs, food or alcohol. Drugs such as aspirin affect the elimination of the uric acid by the kidneys and increase the chances of gout. Acidic diuretics (drugs that increase the formation of urine) also slow down elimination of uric acid.

Caution and Recommendations to Therapists:

Advice the client to reduce intake of purine rich diets such as liver, kidney, sardines, anchovies and sweet breads.

Do not massage during the acute stage. Passive range of motion is also contraindicated. The joint should be rested in this stage. Cold packs may be beneficial.

In the subacute stage, light massage may be done in surrounding areas. Range of motion and local massage should not be done.

In the chronic stages, the aim should be to increase circulation by light to medium brisk massage. However, the duration should be short. Refer to Appendix IV for resources.

Notes: ───

Arthritis - infective (Septic arthritis)

Musculoskeletal system

An inflammation of joint structures due to infection.

Cause:

It can be caused by a variety of bacterial diseases including gonorrhea, scarlet fever, enteric fever, or spread of infection directly from the surrounding area or blood borne from another infected part of body.

Signs and Symptoms:

There is a sudden swelling and inflammation of the joint with the joint cavity filled with pus or fibrinous fluid. In the chronic type of arthritis, healing occurs by fibrosis which in turn leads to stiffening of the joint. The infection may spread to the bone, ligaments and cartilage in that area. The client may complain of severe pain. Muscles around the joint may go into spasm. This may be accompanied by fever.

Risk factors:

Bacterial infection of any kind in other regions, or chronic illness like diabetes, rheumatoid arthritis, increases the susceptibility. Alcoholics and elderly people are also prone. Any disease that depresses the immune system or immunosuppressive drugs puts an individual at high risk.

Caution and Recommendations to Therapists:

Do not massage till the inflammation has subsided. Very gentle massage may be given far away from the inflamed joint. During/after recovery heat application with vigorous and deep massage should be given along with passive stretching.

Notes: —————————————————————————————————————

Encourage client to take the full course of antibiotics. To reduce adhesions intra-articular drainage is done to remove the pus from the joint cavity. This condition is considered as a medical emergency as the infection can destroy the articular cartilage and bone.

Arthritis - osteoarthritis (Osteoarthrosis)

Musculoskeletal system

A chronic degenerative joint disease.

Cause:

The cause is unknown in the primary type. The secondary type occurs after injury to the joint, ligament or cartilage. Excess mechanical stress placed on the joint due to developmental defects or overweight can also produce osteoarthritis.

Signs and Symptoms:

Osteoarthritis typically affects single large synovial joints. It affects joints asymmetrically. There is a progressive loss of articular cartilage and inflammation of the synovial membrane. There is joint pain, stiffness, limitation of motion, joint instability and deformity. Pain occurs at rest and several hours after use. Cracking sounds are produced in the affected joint on movement. It commonly affects the hips, knees, lumbar and cervical vertebrae, ie., primarily the weight-bearing joints.

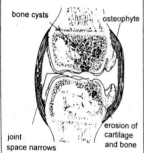

If the cervical spine is affected the client complains of localized stiffness. In lumbar spine involvement, there is low back pain and stiffness, muscle spasm and loss of mobility. There may be pain due to the compression of nerve roots.

Osteoarthritis of the hip causes pain in the groin region or the inner aspect of the thigh. The pain may be referred to the gluteal region or knee. Movement of the hip is restricted. The client may hold the hip flexed, externally rotated and adducted. The gait may be affected. The client may have difficulty getting up after sitting. The muscles around the hip may be atrophied.

In the case of knee, the joint may be swollen with fluid and movement may be limited.

Risk factors:

The incidence increases with age. There is a genetic predisposition in some individuals. Immunologic factors have also been implicated in accelerating the changes in the primary type.

Caution and Recommendations to Therapists:

Deep moist heat application improves the circulation around the joints. Passive movement and friction of the joint are indicated when pain is minimal. Trigger point therapy, lymphatic drainage techniques are other forms of treatment that have been used.

Notes: _____

Arthritis - rheumatoid   Musculoskeletal system

One of the autoimmune diseases that affects multiple systems, producing degenerative changes in connective tissue and inflammatory vascular lesions.

Cause:

It is an autoimmune disease where antibodies called rheumatoid factors are produced against the body's own antibodies.

Signs and Symptoms:

The antigen-antibody reaction that takes place in the synovial tissue of joints attracts lymphocytes and macrophages to the area along with the stimulation of the complement system. In long standing arthritis of the joints the finger, the finger appears spindle shaped.

Diagnosis is made based on a specific criteria. Typically, the client complains of morning stiffness for at least one hour over 6 weeks, swelling of more than three joints for over 6 weeks, with symmetrical joint swelling. In arthritis of the hand, the metacarpophalangeal joints are flexed, the first interphalangeal joints hyperextended, and the second interphalangeal joint flexed. Rheumatoid arthritis can affect any joint, but the small joints of the limbs are more commonly affected.

Risk factors:

It is more common in women in the older age group. There is also a genetic predisposition. Often, there is a family history of the disease. Exposure to cold and dampness are other predisposing factors.

Caution and Recommendations to Therapists:

Arthritis cannot be cured, but it's relentless progress can be prevented. Stress reduction helps muscles to relax and reduce discomfort.

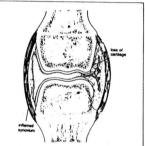

In the early stages the aim should be to prevent contractures, deformity and to maintain joint range of movement. Hot packs help alleviate pain. Massage should not be given in the acute stages, but passive movements of the joints are encouraged.

In the chronic stages, general massage helps reduce stress. Brisk but gentle effleurage and kneading can be used in the limbs. Friction strokes can be used around the joints to reduce the thickening in the periarticular tissues. But make sure that there is no pain.

In general, massage should be for a shorter duration. For clients with this condition, maximum benefit is obtained if the massage therapist works in conjunction with the physician and physiotherapist. The clients may be on pain killers and/or anti-inflammatory drugs that suppress pain and symptoms. The suppressed pain sometimes may result in inadequate feedback from the clients. Care should be taken while massaging such clients as harm may be done to the joints inadvertently.

Refer clients to local support groups (see Appendix IV).

Notes: ⎯⎯⎯⎯⎯⎯⎯⎯⎯⎯⎯⎯⎯⎯⎯⎯⎯⎯⎯⎯⎯⎯⎯⎯

Arthropathy (Neurogenic Charcot's arthropathy)

A degenerative disease of the joint.

Cause:

The degeneration is due to the loss of sensory innervation of the joint and masking of symptoms that follow damage by excessive stress to the joint.

Signs and Symptoms:

There is swelling, warmth, hypermobility and instability of the joint. It may affect one or many joints. Although a deformity may be present pain is minimal.

Risk factors:

It is more common in men over the age of 40. Alcoholism has been shown to predispose to this condition. Loss of sensory innervation of the joint can occur in those with diabetes mellitus, syphilis, spinal cord injury, peripheral nerve injury and leprosy. Recurrent injection of corticosteroids into the joint for other reasons can result in this condition.

Caution and Recommendations to Therapists:

Warm compresses may be used to relieve pain and spasm. Use caution while testing range of motion as the loss of sensation in the affected joint masks the stress that you may put on the joint. A whole body relaxation massage is recommended.

Notes: ⎯⎯⎯⎯⎯⎯⎯⎯⎯⎯⎯⎯⎯⎯⎯⎯⎯⎯⎯⎯⎯⎯⎯⎯⎯⎯

Asthma - bronchial

A reversible, hyper-reactivity of the bronchi to a variety of stimuli, with narrowing and inflammation of the bronchi and difficulty in breathing.

Cause:

The bronchospasm is caused by the release of bronchoconstrictors from mast cells in the lung. The stimuli can be allergens such as pollens of various plants, grass, flowers, feathers of poultry, cat or dog hair, dust mites, various proteins in food such as shellfish, eggs and milk. Exercise, anxiety and stress, coughing or laughing may be stimuli in some people. The spasm of bronchi, inflammation, edema and clogging by thick mucus produce the symptoms.

Signs and Symptoms:

There is a history of recurrent difficulty in breathing and wheezing. Cough with thick sputum is also present. The individual uses the accessory muscles for respiration during an attack. In chronic asthmatics, the chest is barrel shaped, with high shoulders and raised ribs as the individual tries to overcome the difficulty in expiration.

Risk factors:

Usually there is a family history of asthma. Males are more often affected with this condition. Stress and anxiety can precipitate an attack. See Cause.

Caution and Recommendations to Therapists:

Obtain a detailed history - specifically the triggers that bring on an attack. If there is a history of allergy, ensure that the client is not allergic to the oil or other potential allergens in the clinic. It may be advisable for the client to have the required medications close at hand during the massage.

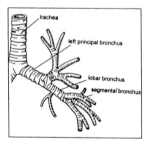

A whole body relaxation massage helps to reduce bronchospasm. The client should be positioned as comfortably as possible. Most often this is a half lying position with pillows supporting the knees, head and arms. Work at relaxing the neck and muscles of the shoulder girdle. Concentrate on relaxing and massaging the abdominal, intercostal, pectorals, latissimus dorsi, sternocleidomastoid and scalene muscles. Massage the muscles of posture - these clients tend to develop kyphosis. Vibration can also be employed over the chest to loosen the thick mucus plugs. A disposable sputum mug with disinfectant may have to be provided. Ensure that the mug is disposed off in a leak proof bag. Deep breathing exercises are very beneficial to open up the alveoli. Ask client to take short inspirations and expire slowly through the mouth four or five times. The expiration should be complete but not be forced.

Consider keeping brochures from your local Asthma Research Council on Remedial relaxation and mobility exercises for these clients (refer to Appendix IV for available resources).

The frequency of massage can be varied according to the client's needs. A relaxation massage scheduled once a week has been found to be beneficial.

Notes: _____

Asthma is considered as one of the Chronic Obstructive Pulmonary Diseases along with Chronic Bronchitis and Emphysema. The best form of treatment is avoidance of precipitating factors. It is treated with bronchodilators, corticosteroids and other drugs that prevent the release of chemical mediators that cause broncho-constriction. Refer to Appendix III for details of side effects.

Atelectasis (Collapsed lung)   Respiratory system

A lack of expansion of small or larger parts of the lung segments.

Cause:

Blockage of the bronchi/bronchioles by thick mucus secretions or foreign bodies causes lack of air flow into the areas beyond the blockage. This leads to slow absorption into the blood, of even the little air remaining in the area and collapse of this segment of lung. The area may become slowly expansible after healing/removal of the blockage. If there is an inflammatory reaction, it may heal by fibrosis with permanent collapse and damage to the lung.

Signs and Symptoms:

There is difficulty and abnormal awareness of breathing (dyspnea). If only a small area is affected there may be no symptoms. If a very large area is affected the ribs and intercostal regions are drawn abnormally inwards while breathing. The tips of fingers, toes and tongue may appear blue (cyanosis), along with a rapid heart rate.

Risk factors:

Any chronic obstructive disease, cystic fibrosis and pulmonary edema can predispose to atelectasis. It is more common in heavy smokers. Any condition that makes deep breathing painful such as fractured ribs, upper abdominal surgery, obesity, prolonged immobility/bed rest predispose to atelectasis.

Caution and Recommendations to Therapists:

Increase humidity and warmth of room before massaging these clients as it helps to loosen thick and plugged mucus. There should be proper air circulation and filtration in the clinic.

The aim is to reduce the symptoms and help with the drainage of the excess mucus by dislodging them from the walls of the bronchi and to increase the mobility of the thorax. Since the basal regions of the lungs are most affected, position the client with the head end lower than the rest of the body either by using pillows under the abdomen to raise it or tilting the table with the foot end higher than the head end. Let the client relax for about ten minutes in this position before massage. Encourage clients to breath deeply with slow and full expiration throughout the massage. Steam inhalation at this point helps loosen the thick sputum. Do a whole body relaxation massage and use vigorous chest clapping, hacking and vibrations for 10 to 20 minutes. You may have to provide a sputum mug with disinfectant for the client. Use proper precautions while handling and disposing the mug and contents. Massage the tired respiratory muscles and the accessory muscles that are used for respiration. This should include the pectorals, the latissimus dorsi, trapezius, sternocleidomastoid and scalene muscles.

These clients are very prone to respiratory infection. Do not massage if you have any form of respiratory infection. Schedule these clients for a time when they are unlikely to come in contact with others with infection. Encourage client to loose weight if obese and stop smoking if a smoker.

Notes: _____

Atherosclerosis
Cardiovascular system

(Greek:atheros-paste, sclerosis-hardness)

Deposition of fibro-fatty substances in the inner lining of medium and large sized arteries.

Cause:

There is hardening and narrowing of large and medium sized arteries due to accumulation of lipids intracellularly and extracellularly. There is also proliferation of smooth muscle cells and formation of scar tissue in the vessels thus producing narrowing. Thrombus formation is thus encouraged.

Signs and Symptoms:

The client may have no symptoms and signs as this disease is slow in onset. They may give a history of thrombosis, angina, myocardial infarction (heart attack), or stroke. Superficial arteries may be hard and thickened. Edema and discoloration of the skin may be seen.

Risk factors:

It is more common in males over 35 and in post menopausal women. The incidence is higher in African-Americans. Cigarette smoking, oral contraceptives, high serum cholesterol levels (>200mg/100ml) with high levels of low density lipoproteins (type of proteins which help transport cholesterol in the blood) increase the risk. Clients with hypertension, diabetes, obese clients, those leading a sedentary lifestyle, those of type A personality, and highly stressed individuals are all predisposed.

Caution and Recommendations to Therapists:

Since these clients are prone for thrombus formation, deep strokes are likely to dislodge thrombus, if present, from their point of attachment. The thrombus can float as an emboli and clog smaller arteries in the lungs, heart or brain leading to pulmonary edema and difficulty in breathing, infarction or stroke. If the client gives a history of previous strokes, chronic hypertension or thrombus, massage should be given only after consulting the physician. Use gentle strokes in all clients with this condition.

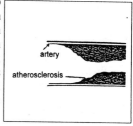

Consider keeping brochures from your local Hypertension Society or Association in your waiting room (see Appendix IV). Encourage high risk clients to get their blood pressure and cholesterol levels checked regularly.

Notes: ───

Bell's palsy

Disease of the VIIth cranial nerve - facial nerve that results in paralysis on one side of the face.

Cause:

It is commonly caused by inflammation around the nerve as it travels from the brain to the exterior. The facial muscles supplied by this nerve undergo paralysis. Pressure on the nerve by tumors, injury to the nerve, infection of the meninges or the inner ear or dental surgery can cause this. Diabetes, pregnancy and hypertension are other causes.

Signs and Symptoms:

The disorder comes on suddenly. The flaccid paralysis of the facial muscles result in drooping of the mouth on the affected side and difficulty in puckering the lips

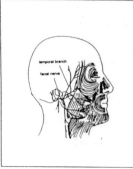

(due to paralysis of the orbicularis oris). If the nerve has been affected proximal to the branch carrying taste sensations from the anterior two third of the tongue, taste is diminished or lost. The person has difficulty closing the eyes tightly (orbicularis oculi affected) and creasing the forehead (paralysis of occipito frontalis). Affectation of the buccinator prevents the client from puffing the cheeks and is the cause of food getting caught between the teeth and cheeks. There is also excessive tearing from the affected eye. Due to the incomplete closure of the eye these individuals are prone for conjunctivitis. Pain may be present near the angle of the jaw and behind the ear.

Risk factors:

Colds and chills have been found to trigger Bell's palsy.

Caution and Recommendations to Therapists:

Stabilise the clients head. Use light strokes from the middle of face to the sides with the strokes directed upwards. To increase the tone on the affected side use kneading strokes with the finger tip. Light tapotement and vibration help stimulate the paralyzed muscles. Active exercises may also be used. To exercise the orbicularis oculi ask client to alternately close and open eyes with and without mild resistance to the eyelids. For the buccinator the cheeks should be puffed out and in. Ask client to try and whistle. For the orbicularis oris the mouth should be puckered. Ask client to smile as widely as possible. Saying words that use the letters P,B,M,N also exercise the labials. To exercise the frontalis ask client to raise and lower eyebrows. Application of moist heat to the affected side may help reduce the pain, if present. Spend about 15 minutes massaging the face. Teach client to massage the face regularly. To maintain the tone, massage can be done two to three times a day.

Notes: _____

Eighty to ninety percent of individuals recover spontaneously and completely in 1-8 weeks. Corticosteroids are used to reduce the inflammation of the nerve. Electrotherapy may be used to reduce the speed of atrophy of the facial muscles.

Bronchiectasis

An abnormal dilation and destruction of the walls of the bronchi.

Cause:

It is caused by any condition that repeatedly damages the bronchial walls and supporting tissues and reduces the action of the cilia that help clear the mucus. There is a collection of mucus in the dilated bronchi. An inflammatory reaction results with further weakening of the walls. The ciliated epithelium is replaced by squamous epithelium hindering the clearance of mucus further. The dilatation may be confined to one or more lobes of the lungs.

Signs and Symptoms:

It is usually asymptomatic at the start. Frequent episodes of pneumonia or blood-tinged sputum follow. Classically, there is a persistent cough with large amounts of foul smelling yellow colored sputum. Noisy breathing, difficulty in breathing, loss of weight, anemia, recurrent fever with chills are other symptoms.

Risk factors:

It is more common in chronic smokers. Men are more often affected. Lung tumors, foreign body obstruction, recurrent respiratory infections, tuberculosis, fungal infections of lungs, cystic fibrosis, congenital malformation of bronchi and inhalation of corrosive gases are other predisposing factors.

Caution and Recommendations to Therapists:

The aim is to reduce the symptoms and help with the drainage of the excess mucus by dislodging them from the walls of the bronchi and to increase the mobility of the thorax.

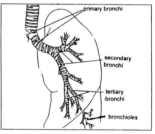

The client has to be positioned according to the lobe that is affected for maximum benefit. The bronchi of the lobe affected should be facing downwards and towards the main bronchi so that gravity could also be used to drain secretions. For lower lobe drainage (most common), position client with head end lower than foot end (see bronchitis) with the help of pillows. For draining the middle lobe the client should lie flat on the back with pillows arranged to turn the body to left or right at an angle of 45 degrees away from the affected side. For upper lobe drainage, a seated position should be used. Steam inhalation before treatment is beneficial. Alternately, increase the humidity and warmth of the room while treating such clients. Use hacking, clapping and vibration movements over chest for 20-30 minutes. Do a whole body relaxation massage. Massage the tired respiratory muscles and the accessory muscles that are used for respiration. This should include the pectorals, the latissimus dorsi, trapezius, sternocleidomastoid and scalene muscles. Encourage clients to breath deeply with slow and full expiration. You may have to provide a sputum mug with disinfectant for the client. Use proper precautions while handling and disposing the mug and contents.

Notes: ———

Bronchiectasis is treated with antibiotics if an infection is suspected. Postural drainage and bronchodilators are key elements of treatment. See Appendix III for details of drugs and side effects. Sometimes surgery may be required to remove a severely affected lobe.

Bronchitis Respiratory system

An acute or chronic inflammation of the bronchi and trachea. It is one of the Chronic Obstructive Pulmonary Diseases (COPD)

Cause:

Many of the situations cited under risk factors result in impairment of ciliary action of the respiratory epithelium and reduced macrophage function in the airways. As a result the immunity is lowered locally. Also, the mucus is not cleared from the airways causing narrowing and plugging of the bronchioles. The mucus also serves as a nidus for bacteria to multiply making the individual more prone for infection. All of the above cause excess mucus production, inflammation and destruction of the alveolar septae. Healing occurs by fibrosis around the bronchi producing narrowing. This sequence of events is responsible for the chronic symptoms in those with bronchitis.

Signs and Symptoms:

Typically there is a history of smoking. The person has cough with sputum and has a reduced capacity to exercise or do strenuous work. Soon the symptoms progress to difficulty in breathing even on minimal exertion. Sounds may be heard over the chest as the air flows through the narrowed bronchi. There is recurrent respiratory infection and the disease progresses, if left untreated, to respiratory failure and death.

Risk factors:

It is more common in individuals over 40. Men are more frequently affected with this condition. Bronchitis tends to recur in winter. Smoking, respiratory allergies and recurrent respiratory infections are commonly associated with bronchitis. This disorder can occur as a complication of tonsillitis, sinusitis or pharyngitis. Cold, moist environment, constant exposure to dust, smoke or fumes also predispose to the condition.

Caution and Recommendations to Therapists:

The aim is to reduce the symptoms and help with the drainage of the excess mucus by dislodging them from the walls of the bronchi and to help with the mobility of the thorax.

Proper air circulation and filtration in the clinic helps these clients. Higher humidity and warmth also helps with the drainage of mucus. Since the basal regions of the lungs are most affected, position the client with the head end lower than the rest of the body either by using pillows under the abdomen to raise it or tilting the table with the foot end higher than the head end. Let the client relax for about ten minutes in this position before massage. Steam inhalation at this point helps loosen the thick sputum.

Do a whole body relaxation massage and use vigorous chest clapping, hacking and vibrations for 10 to 20 minutes. You may have to provide a sputum mug with disinfectant for the client. (Use proper precautions while handling and disposing the mug and contents). Massage the tired respiratory muscles and the accessory muscles that are used for respiration. This should include the pectorals, the latissimus dorsi, trapezius, sternocleidomastoid and scalene muscles. Encourage clients to breath deeply with slow and full expiration throughout the massage treatment.

These clients are very prone to respiratory infection so massage should be avoided if the therapist has even a mild form of respiratory infection. Schedule these clients for a time when they are unlikely to come in contact with others with infection. Encourage client to stop smoking if smokers.

Notes: ────────────────────────────────

Chronic Bronchitis is considered as one of the Chronic Obstructive Pulmonary Diseases along with Emphysema and Asthma. The disease is treated with antibiotics and other drugs to reduce the symptoms. However, prevention of risk factors is the best form treatment.

═══════════════════════════════════════

Burger's Disease (Thromboangitis obliterans)

Cardiovascular system

An inflammatory disorder of the medium sized arteries of the legs and arms which can result in thrombus formation.

Cause:

The cause is not known. The linkage of this disease to smoking indicates that it may be due to hypersensitivity to nicotine.

Signs and Symptoms:

The client may present with pain and weakness of the calf muscles and/or the foot on using it. The pain is relieved by rest. However in clients with prolonged disease, pain may be present even at rest. The skin color may be pale or blue, with the skin thin and shiny with loss of hair due to poor nutrition. The nails may be thick and malformed. In severe cases, clients may have ulcers or gangrenous areas (see Appendix I figure 4 and 15). The arterial pulse is weak in the limbs.

Risk factors:

It affects men between the ages of 25 and 40 who are heavy cigarette smokers. The incidence is higher in Jews. Attacks may be precipitated on exposure to extreme temperatures, emotional stress and trauma.

Caution and Recommendations to Therapists:

Massage is beneficial as it helps reduce stress, improve peripheral circulation and reduce sympathetic stimulation. Keep leg slightly elevated during the treatment. Use gentle effleurage and kneading. The effleurage may be painful due to the dragging of the skin. If it is painful, use only kneading strokes making sure that you keep the hand stationary on the skin and lifting it off the client when moving from one area to the next. More than normal pressure may injure the poorly nourished, thin skin. Avoid areas of ulcer and gangrene.

Do not apply heat or cold to the limbs as the local vasodilatation - without increase in blood flow to the whole limb, can damage the tissues. Heat to the lumbar or abdominal region may help improve the overall blood supply to the limbs by the inhibitory effect of the warm blood from the lumbar region on the vasomotor center in the brainstem.

Encourage client to stop smoking. Keep brochures giving details on the health hazards of smoking in the waiting room. Keep telephone numbers of local "quit smoking" associations handy.

Notes: _____

It is diagnosed using Doppler techniques to measure blood flow in the limbs. As part of the treatment, the sympathetic system is blocked in order to increase blood flow. Surgery may be done to destroy the sympathetics in the lumbar region (lumbar sympathectomy). In severe cases with gangrene, amputation may be required.

Burns

Injury to the skin by heat.

Cause:

Burns can be caused by dry heat, hot liquids or steam, electricity and contact with acids or chemicals.

Signs and Symptoms:

The signs and symptoms depend on whether the burn has affected partial or full skin thickness. Burns are classified into three types according to the severity: *first degree* when only reddening of the skin is seen; *second degree* - where there is blistering of the skin and destruction of the top of the epidermis; *third degree* - where both dermis and epidermis of the skin is destroyed. In the latter, regeneration of the skin is not possible and skin graft may be required. If the burn is extensive and severe it results in loss of plasma fluids and shock. The first and second degree burns are more painful as the pain receptors are intact.

Risk factors:

Occupations that expose individuals to any form of heat.

Caution and Recommendations to Therapists:

Massage should be given only when the tissue is fully healed and can withstand pressure. Unhealed skin looks pink, thin and delicate. Avoid massaging over these areas as it may blister on applying even the least pressure. In burns of the hand, support should be given to the hand while massaging and the joints of the fingers and wrist should be moved very gently. No movements should be forced. Uncontaminated cream or oil should be used for massage. Use frictions or finger kneading over the healed and scarred tissue. Give light and stimulating massage to the rest of the limb above the site of injury without dragging the injured area. In clients with old healed burns, massage can be deep, with transverse friction over healed scars. Do not use violent stretching techniques over joints. Olive oil has been found to be effective in treating clients with burns.

In treating clients with healed skin graft, the principle should be to soften and loosen the graft and improve the circulation. Massage over the graft only after complete healing has occurred.

Notes:

Bursitis

An inflammation of a bursa.

Cause:

Trauma, gout or infection from adjacent structures cause this.

Signs and Symptoms:

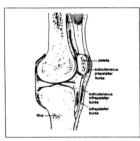

Bursitis can be acute, subacute or chronic. The client complains of pain and stiffness of the joint adjacent to the bursa. In superficial bursitis, pain and swelling of the bursa is seen. Fluid can be felt in the bursa. In inflammation of bursa located in deeper areas, no redness or swelling may be seen. The muscles crossing the bursa may go into spasm due to the pain.

The pain is increased if a particular movement exerts more pressure on the bursa. However, there is no pain in the joint.

Risk factors:

Repeated stress and trauma over the bursa are risk factors. It can be produced secondary to a fracture, dislocation or tendinitis. Rarely, it may be seen in gout, rheumatoid or infective arthritis. It can occur in occupations that involve repetitive movements as in assembly line workers.

Caution and Recommendations to Therapists:

Treatment should be aimed at identifying and eliminating the primary cause. The aim should be to reduce the pain, inflammation and decrease the muscle spasm. Cold packs applied lightly over the area help reduce the pain. Direct compression of the bursa and on-site massage should be avoided in acute stages.

When the inflammation has subsided, massage should be given to the surrounding muscles with friction directly over the joint. Ice packs should be used after friction techniques. Passive movement of joint close to the bursa can be done within the pain-free range.

In the acute stage treatments lasting for half an hour, two times a week is recommended. The frequency may then be reduced to once a week until the inflammation has fully subsided and the full range of motion has been obtained.

Notes: _____

A bursa is a fluid filled sac that is lined with synovial membrane. It is present in the connective tissue surrounding a joint. It functions to reduce the friction that is seen between bone and muscle, muscle and muscle, tendon and bone and bone and skin.

Bursitis can be a recurring problem if the primary cause is not addressed.

Bursitis - iliopectineal

An inflammation of the iliopectineal bursa.

Cause:

Injury or irritation to the bursa by repetitive flexion and extension of the hip.

Signs and Symptoms:

The pain is localized to the groin region and is worsened on passively extending the hip or by active flexion. Both movements put pressure on the bursa. The pain may radiate to the L2, L3 segments ie. to the front of thigh and knee joint and lower lumbar region.

Risk factors:

Occupations involving repeated, full extension or flexion of the knee predispose to this condition.

Caution and Recommendations to Therapists:

Use heat/cold packs to reduce pain. Later use friction massage in the inguinal area. Massage deeply, the thigh muscles and the gluteal region to reduce muscle spasm. Gentle massage over the lower back, thigh and knee ie. L2, L3 segment relieves pain, by reducing transmission of pain impulses to the brain. (also see Bursitis).

Notes: —————————————————————————————

Bursitis - prepatellar (Housemaid's knee)

Inflammation of the bursa over the patella.

Cause:

It is caused by trauma to or fall on the knee, or kneeling over prolonged periods of time.

Signs and Symptoms:

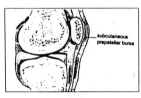

subcutaneous
prepatellar bursa

There is pain over the knee due to the inflammation of the bursa between the patella and the skin or the bursa between the ligamentum patellae and the proximal part of the tibia. A well localized rounded swelling is seen over the patella (if prepatellar) or on either side of the ligamentum patellae. The knee joint may be stiff but there is no pain in the joint.

Risk Factors:

Recurrent stress over the knee predisposes to this condition.

Caution and Recommendations to Therapists:

Massage is indicated after the acute inflammation has subsided. All muscles of the thigh should be massaged. Friction strokes should used around the knee joint and the patella. Passive lateral movement of the patella helps to mobilize this joint (also see Bursitis).

Notes: ————————————————————————————————

Bursitis - subdeltoid

An inflammation of the subdeltoid bursa.

Cause:

It is usually caused by trauma to the shoulder by a fall or blow, or injury to the shoulder muscles. Infection can also cause this.

Signs and Symptoms:

There is localized pain in the shoulder. The pain is intense, dull or throbbing and increases when the arm is abducted. During abduction the acromion process presses on this bursa which is located between the deltoid muscle and the capsule of the shoulder joint. There may be some warmth and swelling over the region. The movement of the shoulder is restricted because of the pain.

Risk factors:

Stress and trauma to shoulder are predisposing factors.

Caution and Recommendations to Therapists:

In the acute stages apply cold pack over the affected area. Massage is contraindicated over the bursa. After a few days, massage can be given with the client in a seated position with the arm adducted and supported by a table or pillow. Start with effleurage and kneading strokes for the upper part of the chest and back. Then use light effleurage for shoulder and upper arm. Avoid areas of pain. Gentle friction is added after the pain subsides. Do not abduct the limb. In the subacute and chronic stage, passive movement should be encouraged. Heat packs may also help relieve pain. (also see Bursitis).

Notes:

Bursitis - trochanteric   Musculoskeletal system

An inflammation of the trochanteric bursa.

Cause:

It is caused by a tear of the iliotibial band over the trochanter. This in turn produces irritation of the trochanteric bursa lying between the bone and the band.

Signs and Symptoms:

There is pain in the lateral aspect of the hip and thigh. It may radiate to the back

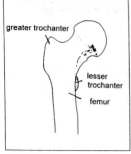

greater trochanter

lesser trochanter

femur

and is increased on climbing stairs, or when sitting cross-legged with the involved leg over the uninvolved one. The pain on sitting is brought about by the pressure put by the contracting gluteus maximus on the bursa. The pain is increased on lying on one side with pressure over the bursa. Passive abduction of the leg also increases the pain. Pain is also produced by pressure on the bursa by a stretched gluteus maximus when the leg is adducted, flexed and internally rotated. However, there is no functional limitation of movement, pain or swelling in the joint. The posterolateral aspect of the greater trochanter is tender to touch.

Risk factors:

A tight iliotibial band predisposes this condition.

Caution and Recommendations to Therapists:

Advice client to use pillows and support at night while sleeping, in order to reduce pressure over the bursa. Climbing stairs or long walks, that can aggravate the pain should be avoided until the inflammation subsides.

Use heat/cold packs to reduce pain and swelling. Later use friction massage over the bursa to reduce adhesions. Gently stretch the iliotibial band. Massage over the gluteal region to minimize spasm of the gluteus maximus (also see Bursitis).

Notes: ————————————————————————————

Cancer- bladder

Renal system

An abnormal and uncontrolled growth of bladder tissue.

Cause:

The cause is unknown.

Signs and Symptoms:

It usually presents with blood in the urine. The person may have frequency, urgency and pain on passing urine. Secondary symptoms may arise if it has spread to the lungs, liver, lymph nodes and neighboring tissues.

Risk factors:

It is more common in men over the age of 50. The excretion of cancer producing chemicals in the urine have been implicated. Those working with aniline dyes as in cable or rubber industries are more prone. Bladder cancer is also common in chronic smokers. Bladder infections, bladder stones also increase the risk. A higher incidence is seen in those infected with the parasite Schistosoma (common in Egypt).

Caution and Recommendation to Therapists:

Consult physician as to the extent of the disease. A light massage of short duration, avoiding the abdomen is recommended.

Notes: _____

This cancer is treated according to the extent and health of the person. Surgery is the commonest form of treatment where the tumor is removed. The whole bladder and adjacent lymph nodes may be removed in some cases.

Cancer - breast

Reproductive system

A malignant growth affecting the breasts of women (rarely men may be affected).

Cause:

The cause is not known. A relationship between levels of estrogen and breast cancer have been shown.

Signs and Symptoms:

Usually there is no symptom. Most breast cancers are detected by the person herself noticing a hard lump. Breast cancer can also present as abnormal fluid discharge from the nipples, retraction of the nipples or as ulcers. Sometimes it presents as redness and increased temperature of the breast. The cancer can spread via the lymphatic system to the axillary and cervical lymph nodes. Spread to the axillary lymph nodes can cause edema of the arm. Through the blood, the cancer can spread to the lungs, bone, liver and surrounding sites.

Risk factors:

It is more common in women between the ages of 35 and 54. Incidence is higher in those with a family history of breast cancer, who have attained menarche at an early age, who have had a late menopause, long menstrual cycles, those who have never been pregnant or have had late pregnancies, those with cancers of ovary or uterus and those exposed to ionizing radiation. Early age pregnancies - earlier than age 20, multiple pregnancies, Asian or Indian origin have a lower risk.

Caution and Recommendations to Therapists:

Refer client to Physician if a hard mass is felt in the axilla or in upper part of chest.

In general, the benefits of massage in reducing stress levels in these individuals is undisputed. Although the role of massage in spreading cancer to other areas is controversial, spread of cancer is also determined by the type of breast cancer (some types spread rapidly while others are very slow growing). Consult Physician regarding extent of disease in those clients who have just been diagnosed to have breast cancer.

Clients who have had surgery that involved removal of the axillary lymph nodes are likely to have edema of the arm. Elevate the edematous arm above heart level throughout the massage. Gently massage arm with strokes directed towards the axilla. Advice clients to open and close the hand tightly six to eight times every few hours. The contraction of the muscles help venous and lymphatic flow. If the client is on radiation therapy, avoid areas of radiation. If on chemotherapy, they are more prone to infections due to reduced immunity. Avoid massaging such individuals if you have even a mild form of any infection. Ensure that these clients are scheduled at a time when they are unlikely to come in contact with other infected individuals.

Notes: ───

It is the most common malignancy affecting women.

Breast cancers are of many types and are classified according to the location and appearance under the microscope. The mode of spread, outcome and treatment varies with the type of cancer and the stage it is in. It spreads directly to adjacent structures, via the lymphatics to lymph nodes, or through the blood stream to distant sites such as the lungs, liver, bones and brain.

It is treated according to the stage. Surgery, chemotherapy, radiotherapy and/or hormonal therapy are used.

Regular breast self examination should be done by all women - especially those above the age of 35 or who are at risk. Mammography - an Xray technique that can visualize abnormally dense breast tissue should be done after the age of 35 and repeated every two years - if above the age of 40 or every year above 50 years of age.

Cancer - cervix

Reproductive system

An abnormal and uncontrolled growth of the tissue in the cervix. (The cervix includes that part of the uterus that projects into the vagina).

Cause:

It is a result of slow changes of the normal cervical tissue into an abnormal type on being exposed to cancer producing agents.

Signs and Symptoms:

It is asymptomatic in the early stages. Later there may be foul smelling, blood stained discharge through the vagina. Low back pain, loss of weight, unexplained anemia and pain during intercourse are other symptoms.

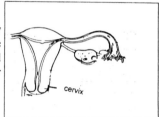

Risk factors:

It is common in women who have had sexual intercourse. It is more frequent in those who have had their first intercourse at an early age, who have several partners, and have had sexually transmitted disease before. There is an association between herpes simplex viral infection and cervical cancer. There is a higher incidence in those with a family history of cancer. Smoking has also been shown to increase the risk.

Caution and Recommendations to Therapists:

Encourage client to have Pap smear done annually, if at risk. Consult physician as to the extent of cancer and type of treatment. If the client is on radiation, remember that the general immunity may be depressed and exposure to any kind of infection should be avoided.

Notes:

Cervical cancer can be detected at an early stage by regular Pap smear tests. This test examines the cervical tissue to detect abnormal cell types. Annual Pap smears are recommended for those at risk. If the smear is abnormal, the cervix is visualized and a biopsy may be taken. The treatment varies according to the stage. At an early stage, just the abnormal area may be removed. In others, radiation and/or surgery may be resorted to. Depending on the extent, just the uterus, or uterus along with the fallopian tubes, ovaries and pelvic lymph nodes and upper part of the vagina may be removed. The survival rate over 5 years averages about 66%. If diagnosed early, it may be as high as 80-100%.

Cancer - colon
Gastrointestinal system

An abnormal, uncontrolled growth of the colonic tissue.

Cause:

The exact cause is not known.

Signs and Symptoms:

In the early stages, the signs and symptoms are vague and related to the location of the cancer. Initially, there is change in bowel habits in a person with regular bowel movements. A dull abdominal pain may or may not be present. General symptoms include loss of weight, fatigue, anemia and weakness. The bleeding causes the stools to be black and tarry. If the tumor is on the right side of the abdomen ie. in the caecum or ascending colon, symptoms of obstruction appear slowly as tumors in this region generally tend to spread along the walls of the gut without narrowing the lumen of the gut. If on the left side - descending colon, sigmoid colon or rectum, the signs of obstruction appear early in the disease. There is constipation or diarrhoea, with passage of pencil shaped or ribbon like stools. The blood in the stools may be red or dark in color.

Risk factors:

It is common over the age of 40 and affects both men and women. The incidence is related to the diet, with a higher incidence in individuals who have a low fibre content and high animal fat intake. It is one of the complications of ulcerative colitis.

Caution and Recommendations to Therapists:

Massage is contraindicated in the abdominal region if a person has been diagnosed with this condition. Consult physician regarding spread of disease and type of treatment if the client is under treatment. Abdominal massage is not contraindicated for those treated with colostomy. Adjust pressure and strokes on an individual basis. The immunity is reduced in those on chemotherapy or radiation. Do not schedule such clients if you are harboring even a mild form of infection such as a cold.

Notes: ⎯⎯⎯⎯⎯⎯⎯⎯⎯⎯⎯⎯⎯⎯⎯⎯⎯⎯⎯⎯⎯⎯⎯⎯⎯⎯⎯

This condition is treated with surgery with removal of the affected part and local lymph nodes (if it has spread) and colostomy (colon opened onto the surface of the abdomen). Chemotherapy and radiation are other options adopted.

Cancer - gallbladder Gastrointestinal system

An abnormal and uncontrolled growth of tissue in the gallbladder.

Cause:

Chronic irritation of the mucosa of the gall bladder can eventually lead to cancer.

Signs and Symptoms:

Indigestion and colicky pain may be present especially after a fatty meal. The pain is located in the right upper quadrant of the abdomen and may be referred to the back, the right shoulder, right scapula or between the scapula. Often the cancer is diagnosed unexpectedly during gallbladder surgery.

Risk factors:

Blockage to the flow of bile as in gall stones, obstruction by enlarged lymph nodes or tumors in neighboring areas can predispose to this condition.

Caution and Recommendations to Therapists:

Consult physician as to the extent of the disease. Avoid massage to the right upper quadrant.

Notes: ⎯⎯⎯⎯⎯⎯⎯⎯⎯⎯⎯⎯⎯⎯⎯⎯⎯⎯⎯⎯⎯⎯⎯⎯⎯⎯⎯

The 5 year survival rate is about 3%.

Cancer - kidney

Abnormal and uncontrolled proliferation of kidney tissue.

Cause:

The cause is not known.

Signs and Symptoms:

There are no symptoms initially. Symptoms of a swelling in the abdomen, blood in the urine denote advanced disease.

Risk factors:

Nephroblastoma or Wilm's tumor a form of cancer with muscle, bone and epithelial tissue is more common in children. Hypernephroma or renal cell carcinoma is more common in men over the age of 60. Smoking, presence of kidney stones are other predisposing factors.

Caution and Recommendations to Therapists:

Encourage clients to see a physician if they complain of blood in urine. Consult physician regarding the extent of disease if cancer is diagnosed. Massage helps reduce leg cramps that is common in these individuals. A light, soothing massage is beneficial. If the person is on chemotherapy the immunity will be reduced. Do not treat if you are harboring any infection. Cross fibre friction can be used over surgical scars to reduce adhesions, if the person has had surgery.

Notes:

Surgery is the preferred form of treatment. In advanced cases, chemotherapy is resorted to.

Cancer - liver (Hepatocarcinoma)

Gastrointestinal system

An abnormal, uncontrolled growth of tissue in the liver that can invade surrounding areas.

Cause:

The commoner type of liver cancer is that which has spread from other areas of the body - metastatic carcinoma. Spread is common from those areas from which blood flows through the liver. Cancer can also arise from the liver tissue - primary cancer.

Signs and Symptoms:

Liver cancer may present as a swelling in the right upper quadrant associated with jaundice or fluid in the abdomen (ascites). Other general symptoms of weight loss, weakness, loss of appetite may be present.

Risk factors:

Chronic hepatitis B infection, cirrhosis and potential toxic agents in the diet predispose to this type of cancer.

Caution and Recommendations to Therapists:

Usually, the cancer is well advanced when diagnosed, whether arising primarily from the liver or secondary to cancer elsewhere in the body. Consult the physician if necessary as to the extent of the disease. Avoid massaging the abdominal area and alter the areas of massage on an individual basis. In any event, keep the duration of massage short. The aim is to alleviate stress and reduce pain. Essential oils of rose or neroli of 1% dilution are recommended for their calming effect. However, avoid use of oil, essential oils and lotions before chemo and radiotherapy. If the client is on chemotherapy or radiation, remember that their immunity will be lowered and avoid massage if harboring any infection.

Notes: ───

The prognosis for this cancer is very poor. The five year survival rate is 1% and most people with liver cancer die within 6 months.

Cancer - lung (Bronchogenic carcinoma)

Respiratory system

A malignant growth in the walls or epithelium of the bronchi.

Cause:

It may be caused by chronic inhalation of cancer-producing air and industrial pollutants such as cigarette smoke, asbestos fibres, uranium, arsenic, nickel, iron oxides, chromium, radioactive dust and coal dust.

Signs and Symptoms:

Usually there are no symptoms initially and it is often detected only in the advanced stages. Late symptoms include chronic cough, hoarseness of voice, difficulty in breathing, chest pain, blood in sputum, weight loss and weakness.

Risk factors:

It is more common in men. Smokers are most susceptible - especially chronic smokers who have started smoking before the age of 15, smoking a whole pack or more per day and smoking for over 20 years. It is also associated with the depth of inhalation and nicotine content of cigarettes. People exposed to asbestos and other industrial pollutants listed under cause, are also prone. Individuals with family history of lung cancer are more predisposed.

Caution and Recommendations to Therapists:

Encourage clients to stop smoking if smokers. Keep brochures on dangers of smoking in your clinic. Have addresses and telephone numbers of local Quit Smoking Clinics handy.

In general, the benefits of massage in reducing stress levels in these individuals is undisputed. However, massage may help spread the cancer to other regions especially if it has already spread to lymph nodes or other neighboring structures. Consult physician as to the stage of disease in individual clients. If a client is on radiation therapy, avoid massaging the skin over radiation areas. Clients on chemotherapy are more prone to any type of infection. Avoid massaging such individuals if you have even a mild form of any infection. Ensure that such clients are scheduled at a time when they are unlikely to come in contact with other infected individuals.

Notes: ──

Cancer - oral   Gastrointestinal system

An uncontrolled growth of abnormal tissue in the mouth.

Cause:

It may be caused by chronic irritation of the mucosa of the oral cavity as in tobacco chewing. Recurrent or chronic ulcers of the mouth can lead to this type of cancer.

Signs and Symptoms:

Oral cancer may appear as a non healing, slowly growing red ulcer or as a growth. Usually it is painful and firm to touch.

Risk factors:

The incidence is higher in men. Chronic smoking, tobacco chewing and alcoholism predispose to this condition.

Caution and Recommendations to Therapists:

It can spread to the lymph nodes in the neck. The nodes are felt as hard, rounded or irregular swelling. These clients are treated with radiation or surgery. Radiation lowers the immunity in the local area and these individuals are prone to thrush and dental caries. Avoid massage to face and neck. Encourage client to stop smoking and drinking.

Notes: _____

Cancer - ovaries

Reproductive system

An abnormal and uncontrolled growth of tissues in the ovary.

Cause:

The cause is not known.

Signs and Symptoms:

It is asymptomatic. Diagnosis is usually made after the cancer has spread extensively. The symptoms are vague and usually associated with gastrointestinal symptoms such as bloating of the abdomen, mild abdominal pain and excessive passage of gas. There may be fluid in the peritoneal cavity in late stages. The fluid can be so extensive that a ripple can be felt on shaking the abdomen.

Risk factors:

It is more common in women between the ages of 65-84. Those with no or few children are at higher risk.

Caution and Recommendations to Therapists:

Consult physician regarding the extent of the disease and the type of treatment used. Avoid abdominal massage. The immunity is suppressed in clients on radiation or chemotherapy. Do not massage such clients when you harbor a cold or any mild infection.

Notes: ──

It is treated with a combination of surgery, radiation/ chemotherapy.

Cancer - pancreas
Gastrointestinal system

An abnormal and uncontrolled growth of pancreatic tissue.

Cause:

The cause is unknown.

Signs and Symptoms:

The person presents with severe weight loss and pain in the lower back. The pain increases a few hours after taking food and is worsened on lying down. If the tumor is growing around the bile duct, obstruction may result in jaundice and diarrhoea. The accumulation of bilirubin under the skin causes severe itching. The jaundice may be so severe that the skin may turn green or black as the bilirubin changes in structure. The reduction of bile slows down the absorption and digestion of fat causing clay colored, foul smelling stools. The cancer spreads directly and rapidly to the surrounding tissues including the lymph nodes and the liver. Kidneys, spleen and blood vessels may also be involved. The symptoms vary according to the tissues affected.

Risk factors:

It is more common in men between the ages of 35 and 70. The incidence is higher in the United States, Canada, Sweden and Israel. Smoking, ingestion of food high in fat and protein, high intake of food additives and exposure to industrial chemicals such as urea and benzidine are predisposing factors. The incidence is also higher in alcoholics and those with chronic pancreatitis and diabetes mellitus.

Caution and Recommendations to Therapists:

The cancer spreads rapidly and massage may help spread the cancer further.

However, often this cancer is diagnosed only in an advanced stage when the condition cannot be worsened. Consult physician as to the extent of the cancer. Avoid the abdominal area if massaging an individual in an advanced stage.

Notes: _____

Treatment options include surgery, if confined to a localized area. Radiation and chemotherapy may also be used.

Cancer - prostate

An abnormal and uncontrolled growth of the prostatic tissue.

Cause:

The cause is not known. Genetic predisposition, high testesterone levels and environmental factors may be responsible.

Signs and Symptoms:

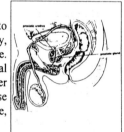

Usually no symptoms are seen. If the cancer is located close to the urethra, there may be frequency of micturition, urgency, difficulty in voiding, blood in urine or blood in the ejaculate. Cancer of the prostate is often diagnosed by rectal examination, where it feels nodular and hard. Prostate cancer spreads usually to the bones and produce bony pain, or cause fractures in the bone after trivial injury. In the advanced stage, as in all cancers, the person looses weight and is anemic.

Risk factors:

The incidence increases with age. It is more common in African-American males. Due to the variation in incidence between races, environmental factors have been implicated. People working in occupations like welding, electroplating, or production of alkaline batteries, which exposes them to cadmium have been found to be at increased risk.

Caution and Recommendations to Therapists:

Consult physician to determine the stage of the disease. No evidence is still available to prove or disprove that massage can spread cancer. Remember that the prostate can be accessed only through the rectum and a massage therapist has no scope of giving clients a prostatic massage.

The prostate is a gland that surrounds the male urethra and secretes a milky white fluid that helps to maintain the pH of the semen and movement of the sperms. The gland is surrounded by smooth muscles which contract during orgasm and expel the ejaculate.

Prostatic cancer is treated with surgery, radiotherapy or hormonal therapy depending on the stage of the disease. Drugs that reduce the effect of testesterone like estrogens are given to reduce symptoms and growth of the cancer. A person on hormonal therapy may have enlargement of breasts and change in voice.

Cancer - skin   Integumentary system

A malignant change in the skin which may be slow-growing (basal cell epithelioma) or rapidly growing with potential to spread (squamous cell carcinoma and malignant melanoma).

Cause:

Prolonged exposure to the sun and radiation exposure are the most common causes of the malignant change in the cells of the epidermis. Squamous cell carcinoma can also be caused by chronic skin irritation and exposure to carcinogens such as tar or oil.

Signs and Symptoms:

Basal cell epithelioma are of different types and can occur as pinkish, smooth swellings with blood vessels over the lesion. It can later ulcerate. Sometimes it appear as thickened areas of skin in the chest and back, that are lightly pigmented. Squamous cell carcinoma appears as a palpable swelling that grows slowly. Melanomas are common in the head, neck and leg areas and usually arise from preexisting pigmented areas such as a mole (nevus). It appears as irregular growths that may be blue, red, white or pigmented (see Appendix I figure 7).

Risk Factors:

Outdoor employment, residence in sunny, warm climates, fair skin and family history increase the risk of contracting this condition.

Caution and Recommendations to Therapists:

Bring to the attention of regular clients, if you notice changes in color, size, shape or texture of preexisting moles and advise medical help. Consult physician regarding indication of massage in those who have been diagnosed with skin cancer as the mode of spread and treatment varies according to the type and stage of cancer. See recommendations under Cancer - breast, for precautions to be taken in those on chemo or radiotherapy.

Notes: _____

Treatment options include surgery, local application of creams or solutions, chemotherapy and radiation.

Cancer - stomach

Gastrointestinal system

An abnormal uncontrolled growth in the stomach.

Cause:

The cause is unknown.

Signs and Symptoms:

In the early stages, the person has chronic pain or discomfort in the upper part of the abdomen. Since the symptoms are vague, this cancer is often not diagnosed till it has spread considerably. There is weight loss, anemia, easy fatigue and loss of appetite. Vomiting is common and often the contents have blood in it. A mass may be felt in the upper abdomen.

Risk factors:

Smoking and alcoholism has been associated with a higher incidence of this cancer. Genetic factors are also implicated - it is more common in people of type A blood group and in those with a family history of cancer. Specific diet and method of cooking (smoking, pickling and salting the food) also predispose to the disease.

Caution and Recommendations to Therapists:

This cancer spreads rapidly by direct spread, through the blood stream and lymphatic system. So massage can perpetuate spread of the disease to other regions of the body. Do not massage without clearance from the treating physician. If the client is on radiation or is being seen after surgery, avoid radiation and/or surgical site. Remember that radiation reduces the immunity of the individual. Do not massage if you have even a mild infection.

Notes: _____

It is usually treated by surgery. Drugs and radiation may also be used.

Cancer - testis Reproductive system

An abnormal and uncontrolled growth of the testicular tissue.

Cause:

The cause is unknown.

Signs and Symptoms:

Slight enlargement of the testis is the first symptom. It may be accompanied by pain, discomfort and heaviness of the scrotum. Soon there is a rapid enlargement of the testis.

Risk factors:

It is more common between 15 and 35 years of age. Those with cryptorchidism are more susceptible. The incidence is found to be higher in those men whose mother had had estrogen therapy at the time of pregnancy. Trauma to and infection of the testis increase the risk.

Caution and Recommendations to Therapists:

Consult physician as to the extent of the disease. If confined only to the testis, a light, soothing whole body massage is recommended. If the cancer has spread get clearance from the treating physician.

Notes: _____

The 5 year survival rate for testicular cancer that has been detected early is very good (about 90%). The tumor spreads through the lymphatics to the abdominal lymph nodes. The prognosis is good even for tumors that have spread to other areas. It is treated by surgery with additional radiotherapy or chemotherapy according to the extent of spread.

Candidiasis (Moniliasis, Thrush)

A superficial fungal infection.

Cause:

It is caused by a yeastlike fungus - Candida. The fungus infects the nails, skin or mucous membrane of vagina (moniliasis), mouth (thrush) or other parts of the gastrointestinal tract. Rarely, it affects the brain, kidneys, and other structures. The fungi are a part of the normal flora which take over when the conditions of the body permit multiplication as in AIDS, cancer, aging etc.

Signs and Symptoms:

The skin may be red and scaly with white colored secretions. A rash may also be seen. Lesions are commonly seen below the breast, between fingers, axillae, groin and umbilicus. There may be reddening, swelling and darkening of the nail bed. Cream colored patches may be seen on the tongue, mouth or pharynx. There may also be itchiness associated with a white or yellow discharge. Men may experience soreness of the glans penis.

Risk factors:

Individuals with diabetes mellitus, those on drugs that suppress the immunity or on heavy antibiotic treatment and those undergoing radiation therapy are more susceptible.

Caution and Recommendations to Therapists:

The fungi is present in healthy people without causing symptoms. Although it can be transmitted by close intimate contact, it requires a favorable environment for its growth. The bodily secretions of the client may harbor the pathogen. Observe strict hygienic procedures at all times. Do not massage if client describes a condition resembling candidiasis or any other sexually transmitted disease unless it has been completely treated.

Notes: ─────────────────────────────────

Carbohydrate intolerance

Gastrointestinal system

A condition where there is difficulty in digestion of a specific types of carbohydrates.

Cause:

It is caused by a lack of the enzyme required for digesting specific type of carbohydrate. Lactose intolerance is the commonest type.

Signs and Symptoms:

The person has diarrhea, bloating, increased gas formation and abdominal pain on ingesting food that contains lactose eg. milk, yogurt, ice cream etc.

Risk factors:

There is usually a genetic predisposition.

Caution and Recommendations to Therapists:

Massage over the abdomen can help release the gas that produces the bloating. However, if the client has diarrhea, massage may increase the motility. In this case, avoid abdominal massage. If the client is asymptomatic at the time of massage, no restrictions apply.

Notes: ─────────────────────────────────

Carbunculitis (Carbuncle, Carbunculosis)

Integumentary system

A bacterial infection of the skin.

Cause:

It is usually caused by the streptococci bacilli.

Signs and Symptoms:

It appears as a single or cluster of pustules that have spread beneath the epidermis. There is redness, swelling and pus in a large area of skin (see Appendix I figure 3)

Risk factors:

Carbuncles are commonly seen in clients with diabetes or lowered immunity.

Caution and Recommendations to Therapists:

It is contagious. Cover the lesion with a piece of gauze and avoid massaging the area with carbunculitis. Avoid the lymph nodes draining the area which will often be painfully enlarged. Wash linen, towels etc. that have come in contact with the client in hot soapy water.

Since it responds to antibiotics it may be better to postpone massage till it is completely treated. Advice client not to share towels, face cloth etc. with family members to prevent spread of disease.

Notes:

Carbunculitis requires oral antibiotic treatment.

Carpal Tunnel Syndrome

Musculoskeletal, Nervous systems

Collection of signs and symptoms produced by compression of the median nerve in the wrist.

Cause:

Any condition that reduces the size of the tunnel formed by the transverse carpal ligament and the carpal bones can cause this syndrome. Reduction in size of the

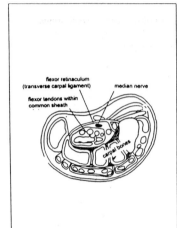

flexor retinaculum
(transverse carpal ligament)   median nerve

flexor tendons within
common sheath

carpal bones

tunnel affects the functioning of the flexor tendons and the median nerve as they pass through it. The size of the tunnel can be reduced by bony or ligamentous changes, increase in the volume of contents as in inflammation of the tendons, edema or tumors. Systemic diseases like rheumatoid arthritis, hyperthyroidism, acromegaly and diabetes mellitus can also produce this condition. Other causes are pregnancy, use of contraceptive pills and wrist injury. Entrapment or injury of the median nerve in the elbow or shoulder (following whiplash injuries), displaced fracture of the distal radius, swelling of the common flexor sheath, dislocation of the carpal bone, vascular deficiency of the median nerve at the carpal tunnel are other causes.

Signs and Symptoms:

Pain in the wrist and hand, numbness of the thumb, pointer, middle finger and half of the ring finger, atrophy and weakness of the thenar muscles are some of the symptoms seen. Pain and reduced sensations are more at night. There is a tingling sensation radiating along the palm if the wrist is tapped (Tinel's sign). If the wrist is flexed over a minute or so, the client feels numbness along the distribution of the median nerve (Phalen test). There may be clumsiness of movements that require fine coordination.

Risk factors:

There is a higher risk in occupations requiring repetitive strains of the wrist by flexion, extension, gripping, pinching movements and overwork of the muscles of the arm eg. massage therapists, secretaries, pianists. Carpel tunnel syndrome is more common in women.

Caution and Recommendations to Therapist:

Since this is one of the occupational hazards, the therapist should take precautions to prevent it's onset by massaging the forearms and hands regularly. Practice stretching and range of motion exercises for the hands, shoulders and neck. Strengthen the forearm and hand muscles using isometric and isotonic exercises. Special exercise equipments are now available in the market. Maintenance of correct posture in occupations which strain the wrist can prevent carpal tunnel syndrome.

On a client with this syndrome avoid local massage over the wrist if there is acute inflammation in the region. In chronic conditions, the local edema can be reduced by lymphatic drainage techniques and elevation of the limb. The limb should be elevated above the level of the heart 5-10 minutes before massage. Deep, moist heat can help soften and allow stretch of collagen fibres that produce adhesions.

Movement of the hand under warm water is another form of treatment. Techniques to stretch the flexor retinaculum should also be employed. Use cross-fibre friction to loosen scar tissue and adherent fibres. Passively move the elbow, wrist and finger joints to maintain range of motion.

The neck, shoulders and arms should be thoroughly massaged. Ensure that the tissue is not damaged inadvertently by vigorously massaging regions with reduced sensation.

Help the client identify and avoid risk factors. Encourage clients to do remedial exercises such as passive stretching of flexors and extensors of wrist and fingers.

Initially, half hour sessions twice a week for three weeks are recommended.

Notes:

In the hand, the median nerve supplies the muscles of the thenar eminence, and the first two lumbricals. Sensations are carried by it from the lateral three and a half fingers and distal part of the palm.

Carpal tunnel syndrome is treated by rest, splinting, injection of corticosteroids or surgery to relieve the pressure on the nerve.

Cellulitis

Integumentary system

A superficial bacterial infection of the skin.

Cause:

It is usually caused by the streptococci bacilli.

Signs and Symptoms:

It presents as pain, redness and swelling of extensive areas of the skin along with enlargement of the lymph nodes draining the area. The bacteria secrete enzymes which breakdown the fibrin network that tries to confine the inflammation to one area. It may be associated with generalized symptoms like fever and body pain ie. flu-like symptoms.

Risk factors:

It is more common in those with lowered immunity, diabetes, or after surgery.

Caution and Recommendations to Therapists:

Due to the pain and swelling, clients will not seek massage. If it is localized to a small area, avoid massage in and around the area to prevent spread. Advice clients to seek medical help and take the full course of the prescribed antibiotic treatment.

Notes: ────────────────────────────────

Cerebral Palsy

A group of disorders that is non progressive affecting the nerves and muscles in children.

Cause:

Cerebral Palsy is caused by damage to the central nervous system of the baby during pregnancy, delivery or soon after birth. The damage could be due to bleeding, lack of oxygen or other injuries to the brain.

Signs and Symptoms:

The signs and symptoms depend on the area of the brain affected. A child may or may not have mental retardation. The speech is impaired in most individuals and there may be difficulty in swallowing. The muscles may be increased in tone - spastic, making coordinated movement difficult. The muscles are hyperexcitable and even small movements, touch, stretch of muscle, pain or emotional stress can increase the spasticity. Due to the spasticity, the posture is abnormal. The spasticity of muscles are also altered with changes in posture for example, if the head is moved to one side, the flexor muscles of the opposite side increase in tone. The gait is also affected. Some may have abnormal involuntary movements of the limbs that may be exaggerated on voluntarily performing a task. Weakness of muscles may be associated. Seizures is also common. There may also be problems with hearing and vision.

Risk factors:

It is common in premature babies, and babies small in size for gestational age. The incidence is higher in Caucasian male babies. During pregnancy, rubella infection, diabetes, toxemia and malnutrition in the mother can increase the risk. At the time of delivery, damage may be caused by forceps delivery, breech delivery, abnormal placement of the placenta in the uterus, prolapse of the cord etc. - all conditions that result in reduced oxygen availability to the baby. Soon after delivery, brain infection, trauma to head etc. can predispose to cerebral palsy.

Caution and Recommendations to Therapists:

This condition cannot be cured but can be supported by a concerted effort of doctors, nurses, physiotherapist, massage therapist and the family. The aim is to reduce stress, reduce spasticity, prevent contractures, improve the posture, improve circulation to skin and muscles that are unused and provide an emotional support.

Since any form of stress increases the symptom, a relaxing massage helps reduce the spasms and involuntary movements. Passive movements and range of motion exercises of joints prevent contractures of muscles. Use transverse friction strokes around joints. Do not use force to stretch muscles that are in spasm. Since most individuals are confined to bed or wheel chair they are prone for decubitus (stress) ulcers and edema in the dependent parts such as the legs or sacral region. The poor circulation in these areas makes the skin very fragile with a tendency to breakdown with minimal pressure. Avoid massaging areas with ulcers and bring it to the notice of the caregivers. Some clients may have reduced sensations. Also, due to mental retardation or speech disorder they may be unable to give adequate feedback about pressure and pain. Use only mild to moderate pressure throughout. Schedule massages once a week or once in two weeks. To reduce spasticity, use rhythmic, repetitive strokes with each session. Initially each session should last for 15-20 minutes. Tapotement of the antagonist muscles help reduce the spasm in the agonist muscle eg. tapotement to flexors can reduce the spasticity of the extensors. Refer clients to local support groups (see Appendix IV).

Notes: ————————————————————————

The spasticity in an individual may change from day to day, with changes in posture and is related to the emotional stress. Keep a meticulous record of physical disability, massage strokes used and duration of treatment for every individual treated, in order to help them maximally.

Cervicitis

An inflammation of the cervix.

Cause:

It is due to an infection by fungus, bacteria or virus.

Signs and Symptoms:

The symptoms are usually low back pain, excessive white discharge, painful intercourse and dysmenorrhea (painful menstruation).

Risk factors:

Cervicitis may be a sequelae to infections of the uterus or vagina.

Caution and Recommendations to Therapists:

Massage over the low back and lower abdomen may help relieve some of the pain.

Notes:

It is treated by minor surgical techniques that destroy the superficial layer of the affected tissue. Antibiotics may also be given.

Chicken pox (Varicella)

Integumentary system

A viral infection which produces skin rashes.

Cause:

It is caused by the chickenpox virus. The virus is transmitted by direct contact, airborne or droplet respiratory secretions. The incubation period ranges from 2-3 weeks.

Signs and Symptoms:

Usually, there is no flu-like symptoms preceding the rash. The rash appears as fluid filled vesicles in any part of the body. Fresh crops of vesicles occur over the next few days. The vesicles slowly become a pustule (filled with pus) and finally a crust is formed. Mild fever, muscle pain and irritability may be present. In those who are immunocompromised the symptoms are severe and may be fatal.

Risk factors:

Exposure to an infected individual increases the risk.

Caution and Recommendations to Therapists:

Individuals are infective until the crusts are formed on the lesions. Those who are exposed to the disease should refrain from work from days 10-21 after exposure.

Notes: ───

The chickenpox virus can remain dormant in the dorsal root ganglia of the spinal sensory nerves and years later get reactivated to present as shingles/herpes zoster (see herpes zoster). Vaccines are available against chickenpox.

Cholecystitis Gastrointestinal system

An inflammation of the gall bladder.

Cause:

Partial or complete blockage of the bile duct and flow of bile cause this condition. The chemical irritation of the concentrated bile causes an inflammatory reaction in the gall bladder. Infection from the gut may spread to the area causing further damage. The gall bladder dilates and swells. Death of tissue can cause gangrene and perforation of the gall bladder with spillage of bile into the peritoneal cavity.

Signs and Symptoms:

Indigestion and colicky pain may be present especially after a fatty meal. The pain is located in the right upper quadrant of the abdomen and may be referred to the back, the right shoulder, right scapula or between the scapula (refer to Appendicitis for location of pain). If perforation has occurred, the muscles in the upper right quadrant go into a spasm. The area is tender to touch. Vomiting may be present. The inflammation causes fever in the individual.

Risk factors:

Blockage to the flow of bile as in gall stones, obstruction by enlarged lymph nodes or tumors in neighboring areas can predispose to this condition.

Caution and Recommendations to Therapists:

Encourage the client to reduce weight and be active. Avoid massage to the right upper quadrant of the abdomen.

Notes:

Cholecystectomy - removal of the gall bladder is the treatment of choice. Since the function of the gall bladder is only to collect, concentrate and store bile, surgical removal of the gall bladder does not compromise normal digestion and function.

Chronic Fatigue Syndrome (Chronic Fatigue and Immune Dysfunction Syndrome, CFIDS, Chronic Epstein-Barr virus infection, Myalgic encephalomyelitis, Yuppie flu)

Nervous, Musculoskeletal systems

A chronic illness characterized by persistent or relapsing debilitating fatigue.

Cause:

The cause is unknown. Earlier it was thought that it was caused by an infection by the Epstein-Barr virus. Now it is believed that the high levels of antibodies to the virus is because of the disease. It may be associated with a reaction to a viral infection in those with an abnormal immune response. This abnormal immune response is influenced by age, genetic predisposition, gender, stress, environment and previous illness.

Signs and Symptoms:

It is characterized by prolonged extreme fatigue. Specific criteria have been formulated by the Centers for Disease Control to diagnose the disease. A person should have 2 *major criteria*, at least 8 of the 11 *symptom criteria*, or 6 of the symptom criteria along with 2 *physical criteria.*

Major criteria - a) new onset of persistent or recurrent fatigue in a person without a history of similar symptoms. The fatigue is not resolved by bed rest and impairs the normal daily activity of a person by 50% for 6 months. b) there is no sign of any other disorder on examination and laboratory investigations.

Symptom criteria - a) extreme fatigue especially after what was considered as a minimal exercise by the person when not having these symptoms b) mild fever c) painful lymph nodes d) muscle weakness e) muscle pain f) sleep disturbances g) headache h) fleeting pain in the joints that migrates from one joint to another, without joint swelling or signs of inflammation i) forgetfulness, irritability, confusion, depression, photophobia, difficulty thinking, inability to concentrate.

Physical criteria - a) low-grade fever b) sore throat c) palpable or painful lymph nodes. These findings should be recorded at least twice, one month apart.

Risk factors:

It is more common in women below the age of 45.

Caution and Recommendations to Therapists:

The symptoms vary from individual to individual and in the same individual from day to day. Hence a proper history is warranted on *every* occasion. The techniques should be modified accordingly. In general, a gentle, whole body relaxation massage of short duration is recommended. The feedback may be inadequate if the client is on pain killers and tissue damage may be done inadvertently by the therapist, so use only gentle pressure.

Refer client to a local support group if available. (See Appendix IV for resources.)

Notes: _____

There is no treatment available as yet, to cure the condition.Treatment is only supportive in the form of antidepressants and pain killers.

Cirrhosis   Gastrointestinal system

(Greek: kirrhos - yellowish-orange, osis - condition)

A chronic disease of the liver.

Cause:

There are many causes of cirrhosis. The most common cause is damage to the liver in chronic alcoholism. It can also be a complication of viral hepatitis. Prolonged obstruction to the flow of bile, toxic reaction to certain drugs, prolonged congestion of blood in the liver due to right heart failure and autoimmune reaction are other causes. Rarely, no known cause is found.

There is destruction, death and regeneration of the hepatic tissue with distortion of the normal architecture. The process results in extensive fibrosis and impairment to blood and lymph drainage with loss of normal function.

Signs and Symptoms:

General symptoms include weight loss, weakness and loss of appetite. Jaundice is usually present. The liver and spleen may be enlarged and can be palpated as a swelling in the right and left upper quadrant of the abdomen respectively. The distortion of the architecture of the liver results in damming up of blood and increased pressure in the veins of the abdomen. This causes fluid to move out of the capillaries into the peritoneal cavity (ascites). The fluid accumulation can be so extensive that ripples can be felt and heard if the abdomen is shaken. The damming also forces the blood to find alternative routes to reach the right heart. One of the routes is through the anastomoses in the esophagus. Thus in people with cirrhosis and high blood pressure in the portal veins (portal hypertension) there is danger of the dilated esophageal blood vessels rupturing and causing fatal hemorrhage. Dilated blood vessels are also seen around the umbilicus and anal region.

The build up of toxins in the blood affects the nervous system producing lethargy, mental changes and finally coma. The toxins (ketones) also cause a musty smell to the breath.

The alteration in the metabolism of steroidal hormones produces menstrual irregularities in women and development of breast (gynecomastia), loss of chest and axillary hair in men.

The deposition of bilirubin under the skin causes the yellow coloration, severe itching and dryness of skin (see under jaundice).

Hepatic failure can also produce edema due to the lack of the protein albumin. The white blood cells are decreased in number making the individual prone to infection.

The impairment of liver function is reflected in various other ways. The lack of clotting factors causes easy bruisability and bleeding tendencies. Reduction in bile formation affects the digestion and absorption of fat and fat soluble vitamins A, D, E and K.

Risk Factors:

See Cause.

Caution and Recommendations to Therapists:

Obtain a detailed history from the client and call the physician if necessary as to the infectivity. If the cirrhosis is due to viral hepatitis, the person may be in a carrier state and can transmit hepatitis (refer to hepatitis).

A gentle full body massage avoiding the abdominal area may be beneficial. Do not try to reduce the edema that may be present in the legs and other areas. The massage oil may help reduce the itching and dryness of the skin. Remember that sensations especially in the distal ends of the limbs may be altered in people with cirrhosis and feedback is likely to be inadequate. These individuals also have a bleeding tendency and bruise easily. Hence use only gentle pressure.

They are prone to infection due to the reduction in white blood cells. Do not massage if you are harboring any kind of infection.

Notes: _____

Clubfoot (Talipes Equinovarus)

Musculoskeletal system

A congenital disorder of the foot giving it a clublike appearance. The talus is deformed and the Achilles tendon is shortened.

Cause:

Club foot may be due to genetic abnormalities. Environmental factors in utero especially in the 9th and 10th week of pregnancy or muscle abnormalities can also cause this condition. It may be seen secondary to poliomyelitis, cerebral palsy and paralysis.

Signs and Symptoms:

The deformity varies in severity, with the worst form being to the extent of the toe touching the ankle. The talus is deformed and the calf muscles are shortened with contractures, at the site of deformity. It is a painless condition.

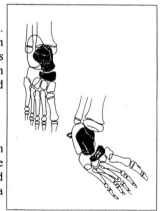

Risk Factors:

It is more common in boys. Family history of clubfoot may be a predisposing factor. It may be associated with other birth defects like spina bifida and myelomeningocele.

Caution and Recommendations to Therapists:

Do not force the foot into a normal position. Relaxation massage with friction movements in the affected foot is beneficial. Thoroughly massage other muscles of the body that are stressed by compensating for the deformity. Work in conjunction with physiotherapist.

Notes: _____

Club foot is easily diagnosed and is treated with corrective shoes or by surgery.

Common Cold (Rhinitis)   Respiratory system

An acute inflammation of the upper respiratory tract due to viral infection.

Cause:

It is usually caused by a virus. Rarely, mycoplasma may produce this condition. There are hundreds of viruses like rhinovirus, adenovirus, coxsackievirus, echovirus etc. that can produce this condition. It is transmitted from person to person by airborne respiratory droplets, contact with contaminated objects like cups, doorknobs and hand to hand contact. A person is infective for 2-3 days after the onset of symptoms.

Signs and Symptoms:

The incubation period is from 1- 4 days. It presents as sore throat, congestion of nose, watery eyes, head ache and dry cough. It may be associated with fever, body ache, lethargy and joint pains. The major symptoms subside after 2-3 days but the stuffiness of the nose may persist for a week. Rarely, complications like sinusitis, otitis media (ear infection), pharyngitis and lower respiratory tract infection occur.

Risk factors:

People with lowered immunity are more prone to frequent colds.

Caution and Recommendations to Therapists:

A cold may resemble more serious illness like measles and rubella (German Measles). If the body temperature is above 100 degrees centigrade accompanied by exudate from the throat, or tender enlarged lymph glands it is unlikely to be a common cold. Educate clients on using other remedies like steam vaporizers and heating pads for relief of pain and stuffiness. Do not massage immuno-compromised or susceptible individuals when you have a cold. Wash hands frequently, cover coughs and sneezes. Avoid sharing of towels and drinks. Consider wearing a mask if it is necessary to massage a client while having a cold. Ideally, the therapist should cancel appointments and take bed rest until no longer infective.

Notes:

Antibiotics are not indicated for common cold.

Congenital Heart Disease

Cardiovascular system

A defect in the formation of the heart that usually decreases it's efficiency.

Cause:

The cause of the congenital heart disease is often unknown. Defects in the formation of the heart may be associated with other genetic disorders eg. Down's syndrome. Some types of heart defects are more prevalent in premature infants. Rarely, defects may be a result of ingestion of certain drugs (eg. thalidomide), or exposure of the fetus to high levels of alcohol (as in infants born to alcoholic mothers) or viral infections in the mother during the early stages of pregnancy.

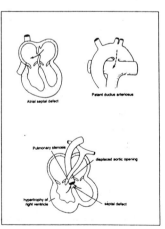

The defects may be in the form of nonclosure of opening between the right and left ventricle - *ventricular septal defect;* nonclosure of the opening between the right and left atrium - *atrial septal defect;* narrowing of the aorta - *coarctation of the aorta;* narrowing of the pulmonary artery - *pulmonary stenosis;* non closure of the communication between the pulmonary artery and the aorta that exists in the fetus until delivery - *patent ductus arteriosus*; or a combination of defects - *Tetrology of Fallot.*

Signs and Symptoms:

The symptoms vary according to the type and severity of the defect. If the defect is mild, the person is asymptomatic. Heart murmurs (abnormal sounds in the heart) may be heard. In some, there may be difficulty in breathing on exertion and the person has cyanosis (blue coloration due to increased deoxygenated blood) at rest or on exertion. Palpitations may be present. If oxygenation of blood is inadequate, normal growth is affected. Slowly, as the demand on the heart is increased, the heart begins to fail - heart failure. The blood that returns to the heart is not pumped out efficiently, and the damming up of blood in the venous circulation leads to development of edema in the liver and the legs. If the left ventricle begins to fail, edema can develop in the lungs (see heart failure).

Risk factors:

Exposure of a pregnant woman to radiation, certain viral infection, drugs or alcohol in the early months of pregnancy may cause heart defects in the fetus. Premature infants are more prone to certain types of heart problems.

Caution and Recommendations to Therapists:

Take a proper history regarding symptoms, signs and medical/surgical treatment. It is wise to get clearance from the treating Physician if the client exhibits symptoms of heart failure. The duration and frequency of massage have to be decided on an individual basis.

In general, a full body relaxation massage in a comfortable position (often seated position is most comfortable), for a short duration is recommended.

Notes: _____

Conjunctivitis Integumentary, Nervous systems

An inflammation of the conjunctiva (the mucosa lining the external surface of the eye).

Cause:

Conjunctivitis may be caused by many factors. Often it is an infection. The infection may be viral or bacterial. In some it may be due to sexually transmitted infections like gonorrhea and Chlamydial infection. The infection spreads by contact with the secretions from the eye of the infected person. Conjunctivitis may also be due to a reaction to chemicals instilled into the eye for other reasons.

Signs and Symptoms:

There is itching, redness, watering and sometimes a pus like discharge from the eye. the eyelids may stick to each other because of the secretions.

Risk factors:

Direct contact with the secretions of the infected individual increases the risk.

Caution and Recommendations to Therapists:

Do not massage an individual with conjunctivitis of infective origin until all symptoms have gone. Encourage the client to see an ophthalmologist if they exhibit symptoms of conjunctivitis.

Notes: ───

Conjunctivitis or pink eye is treated with antibiotic eye ointments/ drops if due to infection. Drops to reduce inflammation are given for conditions due to other causes.

═══

Constipation   Gastrointestinal system

(Latin: constipare - to crowd together)

A condition where there is difficulty in passing or incomplete/infrequent passage of stools.

Cause:

There are many causes of constipation. They include direct obstruction of the lumen as seen in tumors, diverticulitis or intestinal obstruction. Other causes include failure to respond to the urge to defecate, diet with reduced fibre intake, reduced fluid intake and drugs that slow down the motility of the gut.

Signs and Symptoms:

Feeling of abdominal fullness, back pain, loss of appetite are some of the symptoms that accompany the infrequent passage of stools.

Risk factors:

Sedentery lifestyle, prolonged bed rest, ingestion of drugs like diuretics, calcium, iron, aluminium hydroxide (antacids), laxatives and drugs that mimic the action of the sympathetic nervous system are all predisposing factors. It is more common in the elderly.

Caution and Recommendations to Therapists:

If the onset of constipation is sudden, with associated colicky pain, it is likely to be due to some form of intestinal obstruction. Massage is contraindicated in such situations.

A full body massage with special abdominal techniques, is beneficial to those with constipation due to other causes. Massage reduces stress and inhibits the sympathetic system.

For abdominal massage, position the client supine, with the knee and hip flexed. Pillows can be used under the knee for support. Standing to the right of the client, begin with vibration over the four quadrants of the abdomen. Then use overhanded effleurage. The strokes should be in a clockwise direction along the movement of the feces. In order to loosen the impacted feces, use kneading strokes in the lower left quadrant - ie. over the descending and sigmoid colon followed by the left upper quadrant ie. over the splenic flexure of the colon, then the right upper quadrant ie. over the hepatic flexure of the colon, and finally the right lower quadrant ie. over the caecum. This sequence of kneading helps to soften the faeces in the end closest to the anus first and then works backwards. Follow this up by firm strokes in the clockwise direction. In addition, stretching of the colon can be done by stabilizing one end with firm pressure with the fingertips. While stretching the descending colon, fix its lower end just medial to the left anterior superior iliac spine; for transverse colon, fix the splenic flexure - below the ribs on the left; for the ascending colon, fix the hepatic flexure below the right costal margin. Repeat effleurage in a clockwise direction.

In the prone position, massage the muscles in the lumbar, gluteal and sacral region.

Depending on the client, a four week schedule at a frequency of twice a week for two weeks followed by once a week is recommended.

Encourage client to alter dietary habits and consume more fluids, fruits, vegetables and whole grain cereal. Recommend regular exercise training.

Pathology A to Z

The autonomic system controls the motility of the intestines. The sympathetic system - which is stimulated by stress, reduces the motility and secretions of the gut. On the other hand, the parasympathetic system increases the motility and secretions.

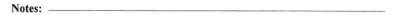

Contact dermatitis Integumentary system

An inflammation of the skin due to irritants or allergens.

Cause:

It is an inflammation resulting from disruption of the natural physiological barrier property of the stratum corneum and stratum granulosum of the skin against entry by foreign matter or organisms. The removal of the fat in the stratum corneum by various external processes reduces the ability of this layer to retain water. It also makes it ineffective as a barrier. In the specific type of contact dermatitis, the irritant is carried through the skin to the local lymph nodes where proliferation of lymphocytes that react specific to the chemical occurs. Thus in subsequent exposures to the chemical the individual develops a reaction.

Signs and Symptoms:

There may be mild redness and edema on exposure to the chemical, with severe itching. It may progress to vesicles or bullae. In chronic stages with prolonged exposure to the irritant or allergen, there is dryness, scaling and thickening of the skin. Secondary bacterial infections may occur in the region.

Risk factors:

A history of allergy increases the risk.

Repeated washing of hands with soap, detergents, exposure to specific chemicals in predisposed individuals can increase the risk. The allergens may include fats such as coconut oil, olive oil, palm oil, fish and whale oil, fat soluble chemicals, perfumes, seed oil, oil of bergamot, bitter almond oil, eucalyptus oil, geranium oil, lavender oil, peppermint oil, rosemary oil, linseed oil, musk, rubber, metals, metal salts, turpentine, gloves, foot wear, oak, pine (reaction to the resin or turpentine used for treating the wood) etc.

Cautions and Recommendations to Therapists:

Always get a thorough history of previous dermatitis and allergies. Keep accurate records of the list of chemicals the client is allergic to. In new clients with a history of allergy or dermatitis, test a small area of skin with a drop of oil that is going to be used and watch for itching, redness and swelling. Wash area immediately and thoroughly if a reaction is seen. Keep antipyretic creams (reduces itching) handy in case it sets off a reaction. Avoid using oils with aroma in such clients unless sure that it will not produce a reaction.

If the reaction is severe, the client may require antihistaminics or even oral steroids. Refer immediately to physician.

Notes: _____

Coxa Plana (Legg Calve Perthers Disease)

Musculoskeletal system

A condition that produces necrosis and flattening of the head of femur.

Cause:

The necrosis is due to the interruption of blood supply to the head of femur by unknown causes. The necrosis is followed by new blood supply to the area with resorption of dead bone and regeneration of new bone. Due to the pressure on the weakened bone, deformity of the head of femur develops.

Signs and Symptoms:

The client presents with pain in the thigh and hip, and a limp that slowly increases in severity. The pain may radiate to the knee and is aggravated by activity and reduced by rest. Due to the deformity of the femoral head, there is muscle spasm and atrophy of thigh muscles. Progressive shortening of the leg occurs with difficulty in abduction and internal rotation (rotation towards the center of body) of the hip. The deformity may be unilateral or bilateral.

Risk factors:

It is more common in boys aged 4-10. There is a familial predisposition to this condition.

Caution and Recommendations to Therapists:

Massage the whole body avoiding use of oil near plaster casts. The oil hastens skin break down and softens the cast. Massage without oil, in and under the edges of the cast to improve circulation in skin. Passively move all joints especially around the cast. After removal of cast, massage all muscles deeply. Use oil liberally over skin that was previously covered by cast.

Notes: ─────────────────────────────────

The treatment involves bed rest for 1-2 weeks, splinting of the limb and in severe cases, surgery.

═══

Cryptorchidism (Undescended testis)

Reproductive system

A condition where one or both testes fail to descend into the scrotum from the abdominal cavity but remain in the abdomen, inguinal canal or other areas.

Cause:

Lack of adequate levels of hormones - from the mother or in the fetus, have been implicated.

Signs and Symptoms:

There is an absence of testis in the scrotum. Occasionally, the testis may be felt as a swelling in the inguinal region.

Risk factors:

It could be genetic. It is more common in premature infants.

Caution and Recommendations to Therapists:

The undescended testis may be located in the inguinal canal and appear as a soft swelling in the lower abdominal area. Avoid massage over area if the testis is present there.

Notes: ─────────────────────────────────

The testes develops in the abdomen in the foetus and descends into the scrotum in the eighth or ninth month of pregnancy. The lower temperature of the scrotum is necessary for proper formation of sperms. Undescended testis can therefore lead to sterility. The incidence of cancer of the testis is also higher in this condition. Hormonal treatment or surgery to locate the testis in a position where cancerous changes can be detected are resorted to.

Cubital tunnel syndrome Nervous system

Entrapment of the ulnar nerve in the tunnel formed by the aponeurosis of the flexor carpi ulnaris near its insertion, close to the medial epicondyle of humerus.

Cause:

Stretching or compression of the ulnar nerve due to overuse of elbow, prolonged flexion of elbow or adhesions cause this condition.

Signs and Symptoms:

Pain, paresthesia and /or numbness in the area distributed by the ulnar nerve ie. medial one and a half fingers is the predominant symptom. The client complains of a dull ache after using the hand. The pain may radiate above and below the elbow. The muscles supplied by the ulnar nerve viz. hypothenar muscles and adductor of the thumb may appear wasted. The ulnar nerve may be thickened and can be felt in the medial aspect of elbow. Tingling sensations may be produced on applying mild pressure to the nerve in this area.

Risk factors:

It is common in people in occupations that involve leaning on the elbow, in manual laborers and individuals involved in throwing sports. Those with a wide carrying angle (cubitus valgus deformity - a wide angle between the upper arm and forearm) are also prone.

Caution and Recommendations to Therapists:

The client should be advised to avoid activities that may aggravate the symptoms. Encourage clients to wear elbow pads. Avoid local massage if the region is acutely inflamed. Passively move the elbow joint to maintain range of motion. Deep massage to the hypothenar and thenar muscles of the hand can help increase blood flow and reduce atrophy. Do not massage vigorously in areas where the sensation is compromised.

Notes: _____

Cushing's syndrome

A spectrum of abnormalities produced by excess adrenocortical hormones.

Cause:

Since the secretion of cortisol from the adrenal cortex is regulated by adrenocorticotrophic hormone (ACTH) from the anterior pituitary, excess secretion is most often due to increased levels of ACTH. Tumors in the adrenal cortex can also produce symptoms. Sometimes symptoms of the syndrome is seen in individuals who are on prolonged steroid therapy for other diseases.

Signs and Symptoms:

The symptoms are seen in multiple body systems. Diabetes mellitus is one of the endocrine problems produced. The muscles are weak and the bones fracture easily. The skin is weak and purple colored stretch marks are seen especially in the abdomen. There is a classical accumulation of fat above the clavicle and upper part of the back giving a "buffalo hump" appearance. The face becomes rounded (moon face) and fat tends to accumulate in the trunk rather than the limbs (trunkal obesity). There is a tendency to form peptic ulcers. The person is irritable and emotionally labile. The retention of water and sodium causes the blood pressure to be increased. Cortisol decreases the function of white blood cells - especially lymphocytes, thus making the person very vulnerable to infection. Since the corticosteroids resemble the androgens (male reproductive hormone), in females, there is a tendency for growth of beard, moustache and enlargement of the clitoris. The menstrual cycles are also abnormal.

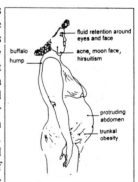

Risk factors:

See Cause

Caution and Recommendations to Therapists:

Very light pressure should be used due to the tendency of the bones to fracture. Do not massage if harboring any infection as the client's immunity is low. Encourage client to take proper medications.

Notes: _____

The adrenal cortex is the outer portion of the adrenal gland which is situated superior to both kidneys. The secretion is regulated by the adrenocorticotrophic hormone of the anterior pituitary.

===

Cystic fibrosis (Mucoviscidosis)

Respiratory, Gastrointestinal systems

A chronic genetic disease that affects the function of exocrine glands (sweat glands, pancreas etc).

Cause:

It is due to the defect in a gene that codes for a protein that involves the transport of chloride across epithelial membranes. The lack of the protein makes the mucus secretions of the bronchus, pancreas and other mucus glands to become viscid. The viscid mucus blocks the ducts of glands, thus producing the symptoms and resulting in other complications. The gene is transmitted as a recessive trait, affecting both sexes equally.

Signs and Symptoms:

The symptoms may develop soon after birth or very slowly. There is excessive loss of sodium and chloride in the sweat making the child susceptible to electrolyte imbalance. The viscid mucus causes obstruction and narrowing of the bronchi. There is difficulty in breathing, associated with wheezing, and dry cough. The chest tends to be barrel shaped due to the retention of air. The person is very susceptible to respiratory infections. The reduced oxygenation of the hemoglobin makes the mucous membrane appear blue (cyanosis).

The increased viscosity of the mucous secretions not only affects the respiratory tract, but also causes symptoms of intestinal obstruction. There may be distention of the abdomen, vomiting, and constipation. The narrowing/blockage of the pancreatic duct can result in difficulty in digestion and absorption of proteins and fat (see malabsorption syndrome) and associated symptoms. Difficulty in fat absorption also reduces the uptake of the fat soluble vitamins A, D, E and K. The endocrine function of the pancreas may be affected leading to Diabetes Mellitus. Other complications include obstruction of the bile duct leading to jaundice and liver dysfunction.

Risk factors:

Family history of cystic fibrosis increases the risk.

Caution and Recommendations to Therapists:

The aim should be to help drain the viscid mucus from the lungs and to increase blood flow and venous/lymphatic drainage in the fatigued respiratory muscles. Before treatment, increase the humidity and warmth in the clinic. This helps to loosen the thick mucus. Steam inhalation is very beneficial. If possible, position the client with the head end lower than the leg to use the effect of gravity on drainage. Massage the respiratory muscles and back using broad strokes. Then use repetitive vibratory strokes. Cupping, tapping and hacking strokes should be used all over the chest to loosen the thick mucus. A cup may have to be provided for the sputum. Handle the container with gloves and ensure that the cup and the contents are disposed in a leak proof bag. Change the position of the client to facilitate drainage through the different bronchi.

These clients are prone to respiratory infections. Ensure that they do not come in contact with any form of infection in the clinic. The susceptibility to infection increases the risk of tuberculosis in these clients. Ensure that you are not put at risk inadvertently. You may have to check with the Physician regarding infectivity of the client if TB has been diagnosed.

Refer client to local support groups and for genetic counseling (see Appendix IV).

Notes: _____

Cystitis

Renal system

An inflammation of the urinary bladder.

Cause:

It is usually caused by infection of the bladder lining.

Signs and Symptoms:

Pain just above the pubic bone, lower back or inner thigh, blood in urine, urgency and frequency of urination are common symptoms. Fever with chills is usually present.

Risk factors:

It is more common in women - due to the shortness of the urethra and close proximity to the anus which harbors bacteria. Stagnation of urine in the bladder due to spinal cord injuries or obstruction to flow of urine as in urethral strictures are other risk factors. Prostatic hyperplasia in men, that narrows the urethral lumen also predisposes to this.

Caution and Recommendations to Therapists:

Encourage the client to take the full course of antibiotics and increase fluid intake. A full body massage avoiding the abdominal area may be beneficial.

Notes:

Bladder stones may be a complication of cystitis. While treating with antibiotics, the predisposing conditions are treated.

Decubitus ulcers (Bed sores, Pressure ulcers, Pressure sores)

Integumentary system

Ulcers of the skin and underlying structures due to excessive pressure.

Cause:

The ulcers are produced in areas which are exposed to external pressures, friction or shearing forces that impair blood flow and lymphatic drainage. The forces compress, tear or injure blood vessels. It is usually seen over bony prominences but can occur in any part of the body. The sacral region, over the greater trochanter of femur, ischial tuberosity and coccygeal areas are more commonly affected. Since, in a normal person, the body position is frequently shifted to reduce constant pressure over a particular area, such ulcers are more commonly seen in people with reduced sensations or in those who are bedridden. It is also seen in nursing home situations where the bed is elevated in one end. This causes shearing forces on the skin as the bone and fascia slide over skin that is fixed against the bed linen. Shearing forces are also caused when a patient with reduced sensations is dragged off the bed rather than lifted.

Signs and Symptoms:

In the initial stages, the susceptible area is red with a superficial ulcer or blister. If the deeper areas are affected, the ulcer has a deep crater-like appearance. Infection may result in foul smelling discharges from the ulcer.

Risk factors:

Quadruplegics, paraplegics, comatose individuals, elderly people with reduced mobility, those malnourished leading to weight loss and reduction of subcutaneous and muscle tissue are at risk.

Caution and Recommendations to Therapists:

Do not massage over and around the area. Recent research has shown that massage decreases skin blood flow and increases the risk of deep tissue injury in such conditions. Perform active and passive range of motion exercises in bed-ridden individuals. Do not use excessive pressure and force while massaging individuals who are prone for pressure ulcers. If erythema\blisters\ulcers are noticed while massaging susceptible individuals bring to the notice of nurses or others caring for the individual.

Since massage tends to lower the blood pressure, clients with severe orthostatic hypotension have to be warned against changing positions abruptly.

Notes: ────────────────────────────────

Pressure ulcers are avoided by constant inspection of skin, protection against mechanical forces, and frequent changes of position in susceptible individuals. Special pressure relief aids such as gel flotation pads, water mattresses, turning beds etc. are available.

Diabetes Insipidus Endocrine system

An endocrine disorder of the posterior pituitary affecting the metabolism of water in the body.

Cause:

This condition is produced when the secretion of anti diuretic hormone (vasopressin) is deficient. It is usually caused by a tumor in the pituitary, or after neurosurgery, trauma to the head or fracture of the skull. Rarely, it may be a complication of infection.

Signs and Symptoms:

Since the antidiuretic hormone regulates the permeability of the kidney tubules and thereby the volume of water that is excreted, its' lack results in excessive loss of fluid in the urine. The person has polyuria (excess urination). The volume of urine excreted may be as high as 30 liters as compared to 1 liter by a normal person. It is accompanied by excessive thirst. The person appears dehydrated with loss of elasticity of the skin, dry mouth and mucous membranes, constipation, muscle weakness and dizziness.

Risk factors:

See Cause.

Caution and Recommendations to Therapists:

Encourage client to continue hormone replacement therapy. Ensure that the client has the prescribed medicines when scheduled for a massage. Keep record of the address of treating physician and other contacts. Massage should be for shorter durations. Watch for postural hypotension and advice client to get off table slowly after massage.

Notes: _____

It is treated with hormonal replacement therapy and surgery if due to a tumor. The hormones are taken as injections or as a nasal spray.

Diabetes Mellitus   Endocrine system

A chronic disease of the endocrine part of the pancreas with inadequate secretion of insulin.

Cause:

Diabetes may be due to impaired release of insulin by the pancreas, presence of inadequate or abnormal insulin receptors on the cells, or the rapid destruction of insulin even before it can carry out its action. Diabetes is classified as Insulin-dependent (Type I; Juvenile-onset diabetes) and non-insulin-dependent (Type II; maturity onset diabetes) forms. Other forms of diabetes are those that develop only during pregnancy - gestational diabetes, diabetes produced by other conditions eg. Cushing's syndrome. Certain drugs that result in loss of potassium in the urine can cause diabetes, potassium is required for the normal release of insulin. Steroids, oral contraceptives, drugs that mimic the effect of the sympathetic system, certain antiepileptic drugs and diuretics can produce diabetes.

Type I diabetes is thought to be caused by genetic predisposition. A triggering agent in the environment such as a virus or chemical toxin, stimulates the immune system to attack the beta cells of the pancreas that produce insulin.

Type II diabetes is more common in people who are overweight and in the older age group people. The cause of diabetes here, has been attributed to decreased number or defective receptors for insulin in fat cells. Also the release of insulin from the pancreas is inadequate. There is an association between incidence of diabetes and family history.

Signs and Symptoms:

The onset is abrupt in Type I diabetes, while slow in Type II. Typically, diabetes is characterized by excessive urination, thirst and hunger: the three poly's - polyuria, polydipsia and polyphagia respectively. The high levels of glucose in the blood is responsible for these symptoms. Loss of glucose in the urine forcibly increases the excretion of water by osmosis. The loss of glucose and water causes the hunger and thirst. There is weight loss in spite of the increased appetite.

The high glucose levels have detrimental effects on almost all systems. Eyesight is affected due to bleeding in the retina. There is loss of sensation in the periphery especially the hands and feet (glove and stocking effect). The effect on the autonomic nervous system results in postural hypotension, diarrhea and impotence.The high levels of cholesterol in the blood speeds up the formation of atherosclerosis with its associated complication of thrombosis and emboli. The person is dehydrated, weak and fatigued. A diabetic is prone to infection and takes longer to heal.

Risk factors:

See Cause.

Caution and Recommendations to Therapists:

Take a detailed history and determine if the diabetes is Type I or Type II. Type I is more serious than Type II in terms of management.

Although not documented yet, experience has shown that massage is beneficial to diabetics and may have an effect on daily insulin requirements. A relaxing and gentle massage is recommended. Ensure that these individuals are not exposed to infections (even mild) in the clinic. The feedback may be inadequate in those with decreased sensation, so the pressure of strokes should be monitored carefully. Ensure that glucose as well as necessary medications are available with the client when coming for treatment.

Encourage client to loose weight and participate in exercise programs if obese. Refer to local support groups. See Appendix IV. Emphasize the need for regular and frequent glucose level monitoring.

Keep a record of the address of treating Physician as well as a contact person. The person may have acute complications like hypoglycemia while in the clinic. Hypoglycemia presents as dizziness, weakness, pallor, rapid heart rate and excessive sweating. Fruit juice, hard candy, honey or any other carbohydrate should be given immediately before calling for help.

Notes: _____

Diabetes is treated with diet, exercise and/or antidiabetic drugs. If severe, or Type I, insulin injections are given. Pancreas transplantation is one of the newer techniques available.

Insulin is required for transport of glucose into skeletal muscle and fat tissue. It also helps store glucose as glycogen. Insulin decreases the breakdown of fat. For protein metabolism, insulin is required for the transport of aminoacids into cells. It also increases the synthesis and conservation of proteins. Inadequate insulin results in high glucose levels in the blood. Normally, the plasma glucose level while fasting is less than 140mg/dl.

===

Diarrhea (Greek-to flow)   **Gastrointestinal system**

A frequent passage of loose, watery stools.

Cause:

There are many causes of diarrhea. Large volume diarrhea is produced when substances in the lumen of the bowel draw water from the interstitial tissue by osmosis. Such a diarrhea is seen in lactase deficiency, high intake of magnesium containing antacids, or when the motility of the gut is rapid. It may also be caused by infections that stimulate the mucosa to secrete water. Infections can also destroy the mucosa and allow loss of water into the lumen eg. Hamburger disease. The infection is most often transmitted by feco-oral contamination or presence of bacteria in uncooked meat, contamination of food, or water and contact with contaminated articles used by an infected person.

Diarrhea can also be caused by inflammatory conditions of the bowel like ulcerative colitis and Crohn's disease. In the latter, the volume is usually small, with blood and mucus. Bacterial infection is another cause of small volume diarrhea.

Signs and Symptoms:

It is characterized by frequent passage of watery stools. There may be colicky pain in the abdomen. The loss of fluid leads to dehydration where the skin is dry and loose, mouth is parched and the eyes sunken. The person feels tired, weak and faint.

Risk factors:

Infectious diarrhea is transmitted by fecal contamination of water or contact with clothes or other articles soiled by a person with diarrhea or food poisoning.

Caution and Recommendations to Therapists:

Avoid massage in individuals with an acute onset of diarrhea until all symptoms have abated as this type is most often due to infection. This is to prevent inadvertent spread of infection to yourself and other clients. Therapists should refrain from work till all symptoms have subsided if they have diarrhea due to infection. In chronic diarrhea, ie. diarrhea lasting for more than three weeks, the cause is usually due to conditions like Inflammatory Bowel Disease. In such cases, massage can be done avoiding the abdominal area.

Notes: ————————————————————————————————

Strict hygiene should be maintained. The importance of changing linen, washing hands thoroughly before and after treating clients, maintenance of cleanliness and disinfection of the environment cannot be overemphasized (see Appendix II).

Diverticular Disease (Diverticulosis, Diverticulitis)

Gastrointestinal system

A condition where the inner lining of the gastrointestinal tract protrudes or herniates through the muscular layer which surrounds it.

Cause:

This disease results from increased pressure in the lumen of the bowel which push the inner lining through the muscular layer - especially in the weak areas. Potential weak areas are the locations where the blood vessels enter the gut. It is most commonly seen in the sigmoid colon.

Signs and Symptoms:

In the more common type Diverticulosis - where there is no inflammation, the person has no symptoms or has mild pain in the left, lower quadrant of the abdomen. The pain may be relieved by defecation. The person may also have alternating diarrhea and constipation. There may be blood in stools. In Diverticulitis - where the diverticula is inflamed, the symptoms include left lower abdominal pain, excess gas formation, nausea, low grade fever and irregular bowel habits. Sometimes, the diverticula can form abscesses and rupture resulting in acute pain in the left lower abdomen along with spasm and rigidity of the abdominal muscles. The reaction to the fecal matter that has leaked into the abdominal cavity can cause high fever, chills and the person may go into shock.

If the condition is chronic, the inflammation and healing by fibrosis can cause the lumen to narrow and produce intestinal obstruction. Constipation, ribbonlike stools, abdominal distention are some of the symptoms of partial obstruction.

Risk factors:

It is more common in the United States. It is seen in the older age group and about 50% of people over the age of 90 years are affected. Lack of fibre in the diet, sedentary life style and irregular bowel habits like neglecting the urge to defecate predispose to this condition.

Caution and Recommendations to Therapists:

A gentle abdominal massage in elderly individuals help regulate the bowel movement. Avoid increased pressure in the abdomen or rigorous massage of the abdomen in all clients in the geriatric age group even if there is a complaint of constipation, as diverticula, if present, can be ruptured.

Encourage client to include vegetables, fruits, whole grain bread, wheat and bran in the diet and increase the intake of water.

Notes: _____

Diverticular disease is left untreated if asymptomatic. If symptoms are present, it is controlled by altering the diet, and intake of stool softeners. If inflamed and infected, antibiotics and drugs to reduce spasm are given. If severe, surgery may be done and the portion of the gut affected is removed and joined with the normal gut, or the end of the colon is opened onto the surface of the abdominal wall - colostomy.

Down Syndrome (Trisomy 21)

A disorder produced by the presence of three instead of two chromosome 21.

Cause:

It is caused by the presence of three copies of chromosome 21 usually due to defects in the way ovum or sperms divide. Rarely, there may be a family history. ·

Risk factors:

The incidence is higher if the birth of the child occurs when the mother is older than 34, or the father older than 42. It may be inherited from the mother or father. Exposure to radiation and certain viruses also increase the chances of having a child with Down Syndrome.

Signs and Symptoms:

The child is mentally retarded, with typical slanting, almond-shaped eyes, protruding tongue, small skull, mouth and chin. The development of the teeth is slow. The bridge of the nose is flat. The person is short statured with short limbs, flat feet and hands. The tone of the muscles is decreased, and balance and coordination is poor. Pelvic bone abnormalities may be seen. There may be associated developmental defects of the heart.

Caution and Recommendations to Therapists:

Massage should be aimed to increase tone of muscles and improve balance and coordination. Encourage participation in suitable exercise programs. Refer parents to local support groups.

Notes: _____

Dupuytren's contracture (Volkman's ischemic contracture)

A deformity of the 4th and 5th fingers due to the shortening of the palmar fascia.

Cause:

Most often the cause is not known. In some it may be caused by a hereditary factor.

Signs and Symptoms:

The 4th and 5th fingers remain flexed at the metacarpophalangeal and interphalangeal joints. The palmar fascia may feel nodular and thick. The resultant restriction of movement in the small joints of the hand may lead to arthritis. Signs of inflammation may be present and pain may be felt on passively extending the fingers.

Risk factors:

It is more common in the elderly, diabetics, alcoholics and epileptics. Dupuytren's contracture may be associated with occupations which require prolonged, forceful gripping of tools.

Caution and Recommendations to Therapists:

If signs of inflammation are present, ice application is of benefit. In subacute and chronic stages the aim is to maintain range of movement in the joints and to prevent adhesions and contractures. Deep moist heat helps to soften the connective tissue before treatment. Friction strokes followed by ice, should be used to reduce adhesions. Use broad strokes to improve the circulation in the muscles of the forearm. The palms should be kneaded thoroughly to stretch the palmar fascia. The fingers should be stretched in a gentle, slow and sustained manner, holding the stretch for 15-30 seconds. Passively move all the small joints of the hand. Resistance exercises should be done to improve the strength of the muscles.

Advice the client to stretch the finger many times during the day. This can be done easily, with the client standing and resting the palm on a table. The fingers are stretched and maintained in this position with the other hand. By moving the body over the arm, the wrist can be simultaneously extended.

Notes: _____

Splinting of the hand, or surgery may be done to release the contracture of the palmar fascia.

Dysentery

Gastrointestinal system

(Greek: dys-difficult, entron-intestine)

A condition with inflammation of the intestine especially the colon, that produces blood and mucus in stools.

Cause:

The common causes of dysentery are infection by bacteria - Shigellosis (Bacillary dysentery) and protozoa (Amebic dysentery). The disease is spread by fecal-oral route and occurs by ingestion of contaminated food or water and contact with the contaminated articles used by infected person. It can also be spread by houseflies. Chemical irritants can be a cause of dysentery.

Signs and Symptoms:

It presents as a sudden onset of diarrhea with blood and mucus in stools. The person strains to pass stools (tenesmus). There is nausea, vomiting and abdominal pain. Signs of dehydration - dry mouth, dry and loose skin, sunken eyes, lethargy, weakness and fainting with reduced passage of urine are seen. Fever may be present.

Risk factors:

The incidence of shigellosis is higher in children, elderly and malnourished people and is common in confined populations like those in nursing homes and mental institutions. Outbreaks can also occur in hospitals.

Caution and Recommendations to Therapists:

Avoid massage until symptoms have subsided completely. This is to prevent inadvertent spread of infection to yourself and other clients. Be aware of outbreaks of dysentery in the local area. Stay away from work if you have dysentery, until two stool specimens have been shown to be negative for bacteria.

In general, strict hygiene should be maintained. The importance of changing linen, washing hands thoroughly before and after treating clients, keeping nails short, maintenance of cleanliness and disinfection of the environment cannot be overemphasized (follow the strategies for infection prevention and safe practice - Appendix II).

Notes:

A mild infection subsides with treatment in 10 days. Severe cases may last from 2-6 weeks. Treatment strategies include administration of antibiotics and maintenance of fluid and electrolyte balance. Drugs that slow down the motility of the gut should not be given as it tends to retain the bacteria and toxins in the gut.

Dysmenorrhea   Reproductive system
The abdominal pain perceived during menstruation.

Cause:

The cause is not known in most cases of dysmenorrhea. In others, it may be due to other diseases like endometriosis, fibroids, pelvic inflammatory disease etc. Increased levels of prostaglandins in the uterus have been implicated.

Signs and Symptoms:

It is characterized by lower abdominal pain 1-2 days before or on the day of menstruation. It is often accompanied by headache, nausea and vomiting. Irritability and dizziness may also be present.

Risk factors:

See cause.

Caution and Recommendations to Therapists:

A relaxing whole body with a focus on the lower back is recommended.

Notes: ────────────────────────────────

Primary dysmenorrhea with no physical cause is treated symptomatically with pain killers like aspirin, ibuprofen, indomethacin etc. (see Appendix III for side effects of drugs).

Eating disorder - anorexia nervosa

Gastrointestinal, Nervous systems

A self-imposed starvation of the body.

Cause:

The cause is not known. It is seen in people who have an irrational fear of gaining weight even though they are emaciated. It is also due to the slim body image being propagated by society as a sign of beauty.

Signs and Symptoms:

The person is usually emaciated and gives a history of inducing vomiting, exercising compulsively and using laxatives and other drugs to control appetite. Sleep alterations, changes in menstrual cycles and constipation are other associated features.

The skeletal muscles are atrophied and there is a reduction fatty tissue. The skin appears dry, blotchy and sallow.

Risk factors:

It is more common in young female adults. This disorder is often associated with depression.

Caution and Recommendations to Therapists:

Encourage clients who have symptoms of this condition to seek counseling and medical help as it can lead to dangerous medical complications and even death. See Appendix IV for resources.

Notes: ────────────────────────────────

Many complications can occur due to malnutrition, dehydration and alteration in the electrolyte levels. The individual is also more susceptible to infection. The menstrual changes indicate alterations in hormonal levels that can lead to osteoporosis.

Eating disorder - bulimia

Gastrointestinal, Nervous systems

A disorder characterized by cycles of eating binges.

Cause:

The cause is unknown. It is usually associated with depression. Many psychosocial factors like sexual abuse, cultural importance given to physical appearance have been associated.

Signs and Symptoms:

There is a history of eating excessively and compulsively. Often high calorie and carbohydrate food are preferred. The individual may induce vomiting due to the feeling of guilt that follows.

Risk factors:

See cause. Parental obesity has been associated with this condition.

Caution and Recommendations to Therapists:

Due to the association of depression with this condition, it is important for clients to seek counseling and medical help as early as possible. See Appendix IV for resources.

Notes: ————————————————————————————

Ecthyma

A bacterial infection involving the dermis and epidermis of the skin

Cause:

It may be caused by Streptococci, Staphylococci or Pseudomonas bacteria. It usually follows a scratch or an insect bite, as a superinfection.

Signs and Symptoms:

It is a deep seated infection with the formation of an ulcer surrounded by reddened skin. It is painful and heals with scarring.

Risk factors:

There is a risk of ecthyma being spread to other parts of the body by contact with it in one site.

Caution and Recommendations to Therapists:

Since it is usually localized cover with bandaid or bandage and avoid area while massaging. Disinfect table and wash linen thoroughly in hot soapy water. If associated with extensive folliculitis or impetigo, massage is contraindicated. Advice client to seek medical help. The lesion responds well to topical or oral antibiotics.

Notes: ————————————————————————————

Ectopic Pregnancy

The implantation of the fetus outside the uterine cavity.

Cause:

Any condition that slows down or prevents the fertilized ovum from entering the uterine cavity can cause abnormal implantation.

Signs and Symptoms:

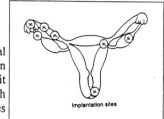

Implantation sites

Ectopic pregnancy usually presents as a normal pregnancy accompanied by slight abdominal pain in the ectopic site. It is usually diagnosed when it ruptures producing severe abdominal pain, with bleeding into the peritoneal cavity. The person goes into shock as a result of the excess bleeding.

Risk factors:

Pelvic inflammatory disease, previous surgery to the fallopian tubes or any abdominal surgery that has resulted in adhesion formation in the reproductive organs increase the risk. Abnormal structure of the uterus, use of intrauterine devices for contraception are some of the other predisposing factors.

Caution and Recommendations to Therapists:

In general, do not massage the lower abdomen in a pregnant client in the first trimester. Avoid abdominal massage in a client who has been classified as high risk pregnancy - this includes a pregnant client with a previous history of ectopic pregnancy. Always consult Obstetrician before massaging a pregnant client who is "high risk". Hypertension, diabetes, eclampsia, spontaneous abortions are some of the high risk pregnancies.

Notes:

The most common site for ectopic pregnancy is the fallopian tube (tubal pregnancy). As the fetus grows it stretches and weakens the wall of the tube until it ruptures. Once ectopic pregnancy is diagnosed, it is treated surgically with the ligation of the tube, if ruptured, or removal of the products if the tube is intact. Incidence of ectopic pregnancy is higher in a person with a previous history.

Edema (Oedema)

Lymphatic, Cardiovascular, Renal, Gastrointestinal systems

Collection of excess fluid in the interstitial compartment of the body.

Cause:

Edema is produced when the net capillary fluid pressure is higher than the pressure between the cells ie., the interstitial pressure. Such a situation arises when there is a) obstruction or reduction of the venous drainage such as in varicose veins, right sided cardiac failure, venous thrombosis, obstruction to flow by an enlarged uterus or tumor, wearing tight garters, prolonged standing or the limb in a dependent position b) capillary dilatation as in inflammation c) lymphatic obstruction as in filariasis, removal of lymph nodes during treatment of cancers eg. removal of axillary lymph nodes for breast cancer can result in edema of the arm d) reduced plasma proteins as in severe malnutrition or malabsorption disorders, liver diseases and kidney failure.

Intracellular volume
27 - 30 liters

Plasma volume
3 - 3.5 liters

Interstitial volume
11 - 13 liters

Signs and Symptoms:

It presents as localized swelling of the area or generalized swelling. Most types of edema are pitting ie. when sustained pressure is applied over the area, indentations can be produced due to the movement of fluid away from the area under pressure. Pain and heaviness of the area may be felt. This is due to the fact that the excess fluid widens the area between the blood vessels bringing nutrients and the cells. The stasis also results in the accumulation of pain producing waste products/toxins in the area.

Risk factors:

See Cause.

Caution and Recommendations to Therapists:

The cause of the edema should be ensured before treatment is started. A detailed history and a consultation with the attending physician can help establish the cause. Generalized edema is usually due to chronic cardiac, kidney or liver problems. Massage may be detrimental to such clients. If the edema is due to causes other than cardiac, kidney or liver problems, massage may be beneficial.

In edema of the limbs after removal of lymph nodes, the limb is hard, tender and painful due to lymphatic congestion. The joints are stiff and the movements are painful. In the case of the arm, swelling may be seen in front of the chest or behind the shoulders. The purpose of massage in such clients is to help lymphatic drainage by forcing fluid back into the capillaries and relieving congestion, by increasing the pressure in the lymphatic vessels and assisting with the formation of new paths of drainage.

The client should be positioned with the edematous limb supported and elevated. Positioning the client in such a way for 10-15 minutes before the treatment, uses gravity to help with the drainage. Use slow, deep effleurage and kneading strokes to the proximal areas and then the distal areas thus emptying the proximal lymph vessels before forcing the lymph from the distal vessels through them. Use friction movements around the joints. The client will have relief even though there is no visible reduction in the size of the limb. Make sure that the strokes follow the direction of movement of lymph in the area. In the upper arms, strokes should be towards the axilla; in the chest, the movement should be towards the neck and axilla of the respective side; in the legs, towards the inguinal region. Use passive and active movements after the massage to assist both the venous and lymphatic flow.

In clients with chronic edema, organization of the proteins in the interstitial region results in fibrosis and thickening of the skin and connective tissue. In such clients, adhesions have to be stretched. Use gentle friction movements here. If there are signs of increased pain and swelling stop treating and refer to physician.

Notes: _____

Emphysema

Respiratory system

A Chronic Obstructive Pulmonary Diseases (COPD) where the alveolar septae are destroyed and the elastic recoil of the lungs is reduced due to recurrent inflammation.

Cause:

It occurs in combination with the other COPDs and the risk factors are the same as Bronchitis (see bronchitis). Here, the recurrent inflammation results in release of protein digesting enzymes from the immune cells causing damage to the supporting tissue as well as the alveolar wall. This in turn reduces the elasticity of the alveolar wall with difficulty in expiration. The destruction of the alveolar wall also reduces the surface area for exchange of gases leading to hypoxia (reduced availability of oxygen to tissues). Emphysema may also be caused by congenital weakness or deficiency of elastic fibres in the walls of bronchioles and alveoli.

Signs and Symptoms:

The individual typically has a round barrel-shaped chest (due to the large volume of residual air remaining in the lungs even after expiration). There is difficulty in breathing, chronic cough, weight loss, blueness of fingers, toes and mucus membrane (cyanosis). The blueness is due to the high levels of deoxygenated hemoglobin in the blood. The use of the accessory muscles of breathing can be seen.

Risk factors:

See Bronchitis. Occupations that involve forceful expiration such as glass blowing, playing wind instruments also predispose to this condition.

Caution and Recommendations to Therapists:

see Bronchitis.

Notes: ────────────────────────────────────

Emphysema is considered as one of the Chronic Obstructive Pulmonary Diseases along with Chronic Bronchitis and Asthma.

Encephalitis   Nervous system

An infection of the brain or spinal cord.

Cause:

It is usually caused by a viral infection. The infection may be mosquito borne, carried by ticks or spread by ingestion. It can be caused by bacteria or fungi too. Other rare causes are toxic substances such as lead. It may also occur after vaccines for measles, mumps and rabies. Encephalitis usually occurs as an epidemic.

Signs and Symptoms:

It presents as headache, fever, vomiting and neck stiffness - similar to meningitis. In addition, there is always a neurological abnormality like -disorientation, seizures, paralysis and coma.

Risk factors:

See Cause.

Caution and Recommendations to Therapists:

Suspect encephalitis or meningitis in an individual with sudden onset of headache associated with fever and neck stiffness. Refer to physician. Be fully informed about epidemics of encephalitis in your area.

Notes: _____

Treatment is usually supportive. Pain killers, fluid and electrolyte maintenance, steroids and diuretics to reduce edema of the brain are some of the measures used.

Endrometriosis   Reproductive system

A condition where endometrial tissue (tissue from the inner lining of the uterus) is found in areas outside the uterus such as the ovaries, ligaments supporting the uterus, vagina, bladder, intestines etc.

Cause:

The cause is not known. However, several explanations have been given. It is thought that backflow of the endometrial tissue through the fallopian tube during menstruation, and subsequent implantation and growth in surrounding areas in the pelvis may be the cause. Some believe that the endometrial tissue may be carried to other areas through the lymphatic system or blood. It may also be due to transformation of immature cells in other areas into endometrial tissue.

Signs and Symptoms:

The symptoms are vague and are usually produced by the cyclical changes that the endometrial tissue undergoes according to the changing hormonal levels in the blood. Lower abdominal pain is produced when the tissue bleeds into the pelvic cavity during menstruation. The resultant inflammation heals by fibrosis and causes adhesions between surrounding pelvic organs. There may be pain during menstruation and during intercourse. Endometriosis may be a cause of infertility.

Risk factors:

It is more common in women who have borne children at a late age. Those who started menstruating at an early age, have menstrual cycles shorter than 27 days, with the menstrual flow lasting more than 7 days, or those with heavier flows are at risk.

Caution and Recommendations to Therapists:

The aim is to reduce the pain. Massage should be gentle and relaxing. Warm compresses to the low back and lower abdomen are recommended. Some advocate the use of essential oils such as lavender, chamomile or rose essential oil in a 5% dilution, to reduce spasm and pain. Oil may also be added to the water used for the warm compress.

Notes: ─────────────────────────────

It is treated with hormones - estrogen or progesterone or a combination of both. Pain killers are also given. Laser surgery to destroy the tissue and reduce adhesions are also resorted to.

Endometritis   Reproductive system

An inflammation of the endometrium - the inner lining of the uterus.

Cause:

It is usually caused by bacterial infection.

Signs and Symptoms:

Abnormal menstrual bleeding accompanied by lower abdominal pain and a foul smelling discharge are common symptoms. It may be associated with fever and malaise.

Risk factors:

Infection of the endometrium is more common soon after delivery, after an abortion, uterine surgery or insertion of intra uterine devices by improper techniques.

Caution and Recommendation to Therapists:

Avoid abdominal area during massage. Encourage the client to take the full course of antibiotic treatment prescribed by physician.

Notes: _____

It is treated with antibiotics that may be taken orally or given intravenously.

═══

Epilepsy (Seizures)   Nervous system

A condition of the brain that makes an individual susceptible to recurrent seizures.

Cause:

Epilepsy results from an abnormal neuronal discharge in the brain. The cause is unknown in most cases. But it may be caused by injury to the brain during birth, infectious diseases that affect the brain - meningitis or abscess in the brain, mercury, lead or carbon monoxide poisoning, brain tumors or head injury. It may also be associated with inherited disorders. A sudden drop in blood glucose levels may also produce epilepsy. In older individuals, it may follow hemorrhage, thrombosis or emboli in cerebral arteries.

Signs and Symptoms:

The signs and symptoms vary according to the type of seizure the person has and the area of the brain where the abnormal discharge occurs. Partial seizures may present as jerking movements and tingling sensations confined to one limb. The person does not loose consciousness. Epilepsy typically begins with an aura - the person may smell something pungent, feel nauseated, have an unusual taste, or have a purposeless behavior. In other types of epilepsy, there may be a change in consciousness with chewing or blinking movements or a blank stare lasting for a few seconds. There may be rhythmic involuntary movements of the limb.

During a generalized seizure, the person falls to the ground unconscious with a loud cry and becomes completely rigid - the tonic stage. This is followed by the clonic stage when the body alternately goes into violent spasm and relaxation for 2-5 minutes. The breathing is affected as the respiratory muscles go into spasm. The person then regains consciousness, with the muscles relaxed. Headache, confusion, weakness and fatigue may be present. Prolonged continuous seizures - a rare occurrence can be life threatening.

Risk Factors:

See cause. Head injury or family history of epilepsy are predisposing factors. An epileptic fit may be triggered by flashing lights, noise, pain, essential oils, perfumes or emotional stress.

Caution and Recommendations to Therapists:

Massage is not contraindicated in a client who has a history of epilepsy. However, make a note in the client's record if they have a history of epilepsy and obtain the address of a contact person in case a fit occurs in the clinic. Since certain types of epilepsy can be triggered by specific smells - aromatherapy can serve as a trigger. Do not use techniques that are deep and vigorous in these clients - this may also trigger an attack in some.

If a client has an aura - a warning that an attack is underway, place the client flat on a couch or ground, well away from hard objects with a soft pillow behind the head. Place a soft object such as a rolled piece of linen between the teeth - to prevent the tongue from being bitten. Do not force anything into the mouth if the teeth is clenched. Turn the head sideways to maintain an open airway. Do not restrain the convulsive movements. Reassure client after an attack and ensure that the client is escorted home from the clinic. Refer to local support groups (see Appendix IV).

Notes: ───

Epilepsy can be controlled with a high degree of success with medication.

Erysipelas

Integumentary system

A bacterial infection of the skin.

Cause:

It is usually caused by streptococci bacilli.

Signs and Symptoms:

It appears as tender, red, swollen areas in the face, arms or legs with small and large fluid filled vesicles and bullae. The client will have flu-like symptoms.

Risk factors:

It is more common in those with diabetes or lowered immunity.

Cautions and Recommendations to Therapists:

Due to the pain, swelling, clients will not seek massage. Avoid massage as it can spread the disease to surrounding areas. Advice immediate medical help. It can be treated with antibiotics.

Notes: _____

Erythrasma Integumentary system

A superficial bacterial infection of the skin.

Cause:

It is caused by the bacteria Corynebacterium minutissimum.

Signs and Symptoms:

The infection may involve one of the body folds such as the groin, axilla or toe web. A superficial rash consisting of redness, scales and hyper pigmentation is seen. The rash is crossed by creases which run in directions different from the normal skin. It may sometimes itch. It is not painful.

Risk factors:

Excessive sweating predisposes to this condition.

Caution and Recommendations to Therapists:

It is contagious. Avoid areas affected if confined to small region, or massage client after it is cured with topical or oral antibiotics. It may require treatment for 3-6 weeks.

Notes: _____

Esophageal stenosis (Esophageal stricture)

Gastrointestinal system

Narrowing of the esophagus.

Cause:

This is usually caused by chemical injury to the esophagus either accidently or deliberately as in a suicide attempt. Soon after the ingestion, there is edema and inflammation followed by ulceration, tissue death and healing by scar tissue formation. Other causes of stricture could be due to cancerous growths or compression of the esophagus by an aortic aneurysm.

Signs and Symptoms:

In strictures due to chemical injury, soon after the ingestion, there may be intense chest pain and excessive salivation. If there is severe damage, there is vomiting of blood and esophageal tissue. Within weeks there is difficulty in swallowing due to the narrowing of the esophagus. In strictures caused by other factors, the difficulty in swallowing and chest pain may be slower in onset.

Risk factors:

See Cause

Caution & Recommendations to Therapists:

Consult physician before massaging a client with stenosis caused by aortic aneurysm or malignant growth.

Notes:

Strictures due to chemical ingestion are treated by corticosteroids to reduce scarring, and antibiotics to combat superinfection. Surgery may be required for severe damage.

Esophageal varices

Gastrointestinal system

Presence of dilated and tortuous veins in the esophagus.

Cause:

The most common cause is diversion of venous blood which normally pass through the liver to the right side of the heart, into the esophageal veins.

Conditions that alter the architecture of the liver cause damming up and increased pressure (portal hypertension) in the venous blood in the abdomen. The blood is therefore diverted through the esophageal veins into the thoracic cavity. Rarely, varicosities may be genetic.

Signs and Symptoms:

The person may show signs of liver failure like intolerance to fat intake, passage of foul smelling greasy stools and jaundice, among others. The abdomen is enlarged with accumulation of fluid in the peritoneal cavity (ascites). Enlarged dilated veins may be visible on the surface of the abdomen. The liver may be palpable as a swelling in the right upper quadrant of the abdomen. The person may also vomit blood (hematemesis).

Risk factors:

Cirrosis of the liver is the most common cause. Alcoholism and liver damage predispose to this condition.

Caution and Recommendations to Therapists:

Consult physician if necessary. Avoid massaging the abdominal area.

Notes: ───

One of the complications of this condition is rupture of the dilated veins with severe bleeding that may be fatal.

Fibroadenoma - breast   Reproductive system

A benign abnormal growth in the breast.

Cause:

The cause is not known.

Signs and Symptoms:

It is felt as a painless, movable, firm, rubbery, round growth in the breast that slides under the fingers. It is often found by accident.

Risk factors:

It is seen in women of the reproductive age group.

Caution and Recommendations to Therapists:

Any lump in the breast should be investigated to rule out cancer. Encourage client to see a physician.

Notes: ⎯⎯⎯⎯⎯⎯⎯⎯⎯⎯⎯⎯⎯⎯⎯⎯⎯⎯⎯⎯⎯⎯⎯⎯⎯⎯⎯

It is not precancerous. The lump is surgically removed.

Fibrocystic disease - breast (Mammary dysplasia)

Reproductive system

Development of fibrosis and cyst formation in the breast.

Cause:

It may be caused by the hypersensitivity of the breast tissues to hormones. It may also be due to unresolved proliferation of the breast tissue due to the cyclical hormonal changes. It is believed by some to be a precursor of cancerous changes in the breast.

Signs and Symptoms:

It is felt as multiple small lumps that are prominent and painful just before menstruation. The lumps may produce heaviness in some while in others it may be very painful.

Risk factors:

It is seen in women of the reproductive age group.

Caution and Recommendations to Therapists:

Any lump/s in the breasts should be investigated and cancer should be ruled out. Encourage client to see a physician. For clients diagnosed with this condition, heat or cold therapy may be beneficial. Use warm or cold packs wrapped in a towel.

Notes: _____

It is treated with pain killers.

Fibroid (Leiomyoma, Myoma, Fibromyoma)

Reproductive system

An abnormal growth of the smooth muscles of the uterus.

Cause:

The cause is not known. Estrogen and progesterone levels have been implicated in altering the growth of the tumor.

Signs and Symptoms:

The symptoms and signs will depend on the location of the fibroid ie. whether it is on the surface, in the muscle or under the inner lining of the uterus. Most often it is asymptomatic. Swelling in the lower abdomen, interference with passing urine, are some of the symptoms. Abnormal menstrual bleeding, premature labour, recurrent abortions are other symptoms that have been associated with leiomyomas.

Risk factors:

It is common over the age of 35. The incidence is higher in Afro-Americans.

Caution and Recommendations to Therapists:

Do not massage the lower abdominal area. Refer to a physician if the lower abdominal swelling is prominent. Encourage client to take iron supplements if anemic, due to excessive bleeding.

Notes: _____

Myomas are treated surgically or non surgically, according to the size and location of tumor, age of person, pregnancy status and desire for children.

Fibromyalgia (Fibrositis)

Musculoskeletal system

A chronic condition that produces musculoskeletal pain.

Cause:

The cause is not known. It has been postulated that it may be due to a disturbance of normal stages of sleep. Psychological disorders, muscle abnormalities and autonomic dysfunction may play a part in this condition. Emotional stress, trauma, surgery, disease of the thyroid have been implicated in triggering the symptoms.

Signs and Symptoms:

The symptoms vary from individual to individual and changes in the same

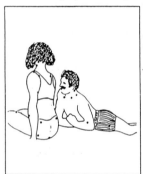

individual from day to day. It is characterized by diffuse, ill defined muscle pain, stiffness, easy fatiguability and disturbed sleep. There is generalized ache and stiffness. There may be stiffness of joints and a feeling of swollen joints although there are no visible signs of swelling. The stiffness may be more in the morning. The client complains of exhaustion and wakes up tired. The symptoms may be precipitated or increased by stress, cold weather and exertion.

It is diagnosed by the presence of tender sites which are constant in location. The common locations of tender sites are bilaterally over the suboccipital muscle insertion at the base of the skull, the anterior aspect of the intertranverse process spaces at C5-C7, the midpoint of the upper border of the trapezius, above the scapular spine near the medial border of the scapula, the second costochondral junction, the lateral epicondyle, the upper outer quadrant of the buttock, the posterior aspect of the trochanteric prominence, and the medial fat pad of the knee.

According to the American College of Rheumatology, diagnosis is made if there is diffuse muscular pain along with 11 of the 18 tender points described.

Risk factors:

It is common in women between the ages of 25-45 years of age. It may be associated with rheumatoid arthritis, migraine headache, irritable bowel syndrome or other connective tissue diseases.

Caution and Recommendations to Therapists:

A detailed history should be obtained every time the client visits, as the symptoms vary from day to day, and the massage techniques varied accordingly. In general, a full body relaxation massage of short duration is indicated. The client may be on pain killers that depress the sensations and inadequate feedback may be given. All strokes should be gentle and rhythmic. The frequency and duration of massage should be individualized. Refer client to local support groups (see Appendix IV for resources.

Notes: _____

The treatment is symptomatic. Massage, acupressure, acupuncture, injection of tender sites with steroids, anti-inflammatory drugs, and antidepressants are some of the treatment options.

Filariasis (Elephantiasis)   Lymphatic system

A disease of the lymphatic system caused by the filarial parasite.

Cause:

It is caused by obstruction to lymphatic flow by long, threadlike filarial worms whose larvae are injected into the blood stream by mosquitos.

Signs and Symptoms:

It presents as a slow onset of swelling and heaviness of a limb, scrotum or labia accompanied by fever. The swelling persists even after treatment, and lasts for years. Legs may appear as large as an elephant's- thus its name. Prolonged accumulation of protein and fluid in the interstitial fluid compartment (area between the cells) causes thickening of skin in the region.

Risk factors:

It is more common in those living in tropical countries where this condition is endemic.

Caution and Recommendations to Therapists:

It is not contagious as it is transmitted by infected mosquitos.

Massage helps push toxins and fluid back into the capillaries and lymphatic pathways not obstructed, thus relieving or reducing aches in the affected part. The swelling may not be visibly reduced, but massage has definite beneficial effects on the client.

Notes: _____

It is treated medically by drugs. If the swelling is extensive and disfiguring surgery is done.

Folliculitis

Integumentary system

A bacterial infection of the hair follicles of the skin.

Cause:

It is usually caused by the bacteria staphylococcus aureus. It may be caused by other organisms particularly when associated with immersion in contaminated warm water eg. in swimming pools or jacuzzis.

Signs and Symptoms:

It appears as a small pustule at the base of a hair follicle. There is redness, swelling and pain around the hair follicle. It is more commonly seen in the thighs, lower legs, arms, face and scalp.

Risk factors:

Occlusion of follicles, trauma eg. hair removal, topical corticosteroids, prolonged antibiotic therapy are all risk factors.

Caution and Recommendations to Therapists:

Since it is very localized, avoid massaging the area with folliculitis. Cover area with a band aid or bandage. Often the folliculitis disappears without treatment. Local application of antibiotic lotions help. Occasionally, it may spread to other regions - when it will require oral antibiotics. It has to be distinguished from non infectious conditions such as pustular psoriasis and acne rosacea. Disinfect table, towels and other linen after treating the infected client. Frequently change the water used for heating hot packs etc. to avoid this being a source of bacteria.

Notes: _____

Fractures

The interruption to the continuity of bone.

Cause:

Sudden application of force that is more than what the bone can withstand is the most common cause. Fractures may also be caused by overuse injury (stress fracture). Pathological fractures occur in bones weakened by tumors or other diseases.

Signs and Symptoms:

Inflammation with it's characteristic redness, pain, swelling and loss of function, is seen in the area of fracture. It may be accompanied by abnormal movement, grating sounds (crepitus) and deformity. The bone may be shortened, abnormally rotated or angulated. If the fracture is compound with the skin open to the exterior, bleeding occurs. Soon after the fracture the local area become numb from a few minutes to an hour, and the muscles around the fracture loose their tone.

Symptoms and signs of complications such as compartment syndrome, fat emboli, impaired healing - delayed union, malunion or nonunion may be present. Compartment syndrome is produced when there is a rise in pressure in a confined area of the body that alters blood flow to the region and affects the function of the nerves and muscles in the area. Abnormal sensation like tingling, loss of sensation, severe pain, loss of motor control are some of the symptoms. Fat emboli may present as disorientation or changes in behavior immediately after or up to a week after fracture, if the emboli is lodged in the cerebral circulation. If in the respiratory circulation, difficulty in breathing, rapid heart rate and pain behind the sternum may be present.

If the healing is impaired, the client may have abnormal mobility even after the normal healing period (4-6 weeks in children, 6-8 weeks in adolescence, 10 to18 weeks in adults). Deformity may be seen in malunion. In non union, abnormal mobility, pain on exerting pressure, loss of range of motion and atrophy of surrounding muscles are seen. Adhesions, and persistent edema are other complications of fractures.

Risk Factors:

Stress fractures are common in occupations that require overuse of one bone. Pathological fractures are common in local areas weakened by infection, cysts or tumors. Generalized diseases like osteoporosis, Paget's disease or tumors that have spread to the bone from other areas predispose to pathological fractures.

Caution and Recommendations to Therapists:

Fractures are treated by reduction, immobilization, preservation and restoration of function (rehabilitation). Massage therapy can play a positive role during the period of immobilization and rehabilitation.

The time needed for healing varies in different bones and has to be taken into consideration while treating clients. Healing time depends on the thickness of the bone, blood supply, amount of separation between the bone fragments, part of the bone fractured, age of client, nutrition, degree of immobilization, infection and extent of bone death.

In adults, it takes approximately 6 weeks in the upper limb and 12 weeks in the lower limb for consolidation to occur in spiral fractures. It takes 12 weeks in upper limb and 24 weeks in lower limb for transverse fracture to consolidate.

During the immobilization period, the aim of massage is to maintain circulation, joint mobility and muscle power and to reduce edema without slowing or preventing healing. Another role is to watch for complications and report to physician. The affected limb can be elevated to improve drainage. During the period of immobilization, use hot packs to improve circulation, decrease spasm and reduce pain in the muscles close to the immobilized part. Passively move all joints not fixed by plaster. This helps the venous return and prevents stiffness. However, do not use forced movements. A whole body gentle, relaxation massage helps reduce the general stress level of client. Massaging around the immobilized fracture site helps reduce edema, relieve pain and tension in the muscles. The massage should be gentle and rhythmic. Avoid the fracture site and take care not to disturb the repair process thus leading to delayed or nonunion. Oil should not be used close to the plaster cast as it can soften the cast.

During rehabilitation, the aim is to help client regain mobility of the previously immobilized or restricted joints. Assess the range of motion of joint and compare with the sound joint. The tissue that was under the cast is likely to be fragile and weak. Muscle atrophy will be present too. Avoid testing for range of motion and tone for at least a week after removal of cast. Remember that although union may have occurred in the bone, consolidation/remodelling may not be complete. In some cases this may take from 6 moths to a year. Therefore, care must be taken not to put undue pressure over the fracture site. Heat packs can be used to help improve circulation and relieve pain. The part may be immersed in warm water before massage. Use friction strokes around joints and passively move all joints. Active assisted movements can be used after consultation with physiotherapist or physician.

One to two treatments a week during the immobilization period, increased to three times a week after removal of cast for two weeks are recommended. This may be followed by massages once a week for as long as required.

Notes: _____

Fractures may be *spiral, transverse* or oblique according to the type and direction of stress. It is classified as *open/compound* if it is associated with broken skin or closed if the skin is intact. It is considered as *comminuted* if the bone is broken to more than one piece, *compression type* if two bones are crushed together or *impacted* type if the bones are wedged together. The rate of healing and chances of complications vary according to the type of fracture.

Fungal infections (Mycosis - systemic Pneumocystosis, Aspergillosis, Mucormycosis, Systemic candidosis)

Respiratory system

It includes infections caused by different fungi.

Cause:

Fungal infections may affect previously healthy individuals or those whose immunity has been lowered. Fungal infections affecting healthy individuals include Histoplasmosis (Ohio Valley disease, Central Mississippi Valley disease, Appalachian Mountain disease, Darling's disease), Blastomycosis (North American blastomycosis, Gilchrist's disease), Cryptococcosis (Torulosis, European blastomycosis), Para coccidioidomycosis (Valley fever, San Joaquin Valley fever). Those fungal infections that typically affect people with lowered immunity are Aspergillosis, Candidiasis to name a few.

Signs and Symptoms:

Symptoms vary according to the disease. Often the symptoms resemble that of tuberculosis with fever, cough, difficulty in breathing, lethargy, weight loss and fatigue.

Risk factors:

Immunocompromised individuals with diseases such as AIDS, lymphoma, leukemia, diabetics or malnutrition are at high risk. Healthy individuals in occupations with potential to inhale fungal spores in feces of birds, bats or soil contaminated by feces (near barns, caves, under bridges, farms) are also at risk. Some forms of fungi spread through broken skin from soil, wood, moss and decaying vegetables and are common in gardeners and horticulturists working with bare hands.

Caution and Recommendations to Therapists:

Avoid harboring caged birds for ornamental purposes in clinic area. Keep clinic area well lit - preferably with natural light, and low humidity to inhibit fungal growth. There is risk of contracting fungal infection through inhalation of spores from dressings or casts. Do not massage until an infected individual has been treated fully.

Notes: ——

Furunculitis (Furuncles, Furunculosis, Boil)

A bacterial infection of the skin.

Cause:

It is usually caused by staphylococcus bacteria.

Signs and Symptoms:

It appears as a large pustule in the base of a hair follicle. There is redness, swelling and pus around the hair follicle. The fully formed furuncle "points" and discharges pus. Occasionally, it may spread to other regions - when it will require oral antibiotics.

Risk factors:

Diabetes mellitus, immunodeficiency, close contact with people who are carriers of the bacteria are all risk factors.

Caution and Recommendations to Therapists:

It is very localized so avoid massaging the area with furunculitis. Cover area with a large bandaid or bandage. The lymph nodes draining the area will often be painfully enlarged. Avoid massaging over the lymph nodes.

If the therapist is affected by recurrent folliculitis or impetigo it should be ensured that she/he is not a carrier of such bacteria, by visiting a physician and getting swabs taken from nose, perineal and axillary areas.

Notes: ——

Local application of antibiotic lotions may help in the early stages. A furuncle may require surgical incision and drainage, if large.

Gall stones (Cholelithiasis)   Gastrointestinal system

Stones in the gall bladder.

Cause:

Changes in the composition of bile cause cholesterol and/or bilirubin to precipitate and form stones. Stagnation of bile, and inflammation of the gall bladder that increase the concentration of bile, also promote stone formation.

Signs and Symptoms:

Most people are asymptomatic. Indigestion and colicky pain may be present. The pain is located in the right upper quadrant of the abdomen and may be referred to the back, the right shoulder, right scapula or between the scapula. (Refer to Appendicitis for location of referred pain).

Risk factors:

Gall stones are more common in obese women of the older age group who have had many children and are on contraceptives (Fat, Forty, Fertile, Female). All these factors increase the excretion of cholesterol into bile. The higher incidence of gall stones in Native Americans indicates a genetic predisposition. Diabetes mellitus, by increasing cholesterol excretion predisposes a person to stone formation in the gall bladder. Conditions that increase the rate of destruction of red blood cells also predispose to bilirubin stones by increasing the excretion of bilirubin in the bile (see Jaundice: Notes).

Caution and Recommendations to Therapists:

Encourage client to reduce weight and be active. Avoid massage to the right upper quadrant of the abdomen.

Notes:

The gall bladder is pear shaped and located just below the liver. The cystic duct connects it to the common bile duct which in turn opens into the duodenum. The gall bladder can hold 20-50 ml. of bile and serves to collect, concentrate and store bile. When food, especially of high fat content, enters the intestines the muscles of the gall bladder contract. The contraction is brought about mainly by secretion of local hormones.

This condition is treated by surgery where the gall bladder is removed.

Ganglion

A cystic enlargement of the synovial membrane

Cause:

It is a separation of small sacs of synovial membrane from the synovial sheaths of tendon or joints. The sacs are filled with synovial fluid. There is a danger of these sacs getting inflamed.

Signs and Symptoms:

Ganglion presents as a rounded swelling, very small or the size of a walnut, usually over the dorsum of the hand or foot, or on the outer side of the knee. An ache may be present over the swelling when using the part extensively. Usually it produces no symptoms.

Risk factors:

Injury to tendon or joints may predispose to this.

Caution and Recommendations to Therapists:

No special precautions have to be taken as they are painless. If surgery is done, massage the arm, hand and around the ganglion site postoperatively.

Notes:

It is often excised by physicians, but it may recur. Sometimes sclerosing agents are used to treat it.

The term ganglion also refers to a collection of nerve cell bodies eg. dorsal root ganglion.

Gastroesophageal reflux

The backflow of the contents of the stomach or duodenum into the esophagus.

Cause:

Dysfunction of the sphincter in the lower part of the esophagus or excessive pressure in the stomach can cause this.

Signs and Symptoms:

The person may have no symptoms. Some individuals may present with a burning sensation behind the sternum which increases on exercising, lying down or bending. The pain is relieved by sitting up or with use of antacids. The pain may be referred to the neck, jaw and arms resembling anginal pain. Rarely, the contents of the stomach may regurgitate into the mouth in the middle of the night, awakening the individual with choking and coughing. Complications such as spasm of the lower end of the esophagus and difficulty in swallowing may result. If the contents regurgitate into the respiratory tract the person may have lung infection.

Risk factors:

Surgery to the stomach, prolonged nasogastric intubation, alcohol, cigarette smoking, use of drugs that affect the autonomic system, hiatal hernia, positions and conditions that increase the intra-abdominal pressure are all predisposing factors.

Diets high in fat, whole milk, orange juice, chocolate and tomatoes tend to lower the pressure of the lower esophageal sphincter, while protein, carbohydrate and nonfat milk increase the pressure.

Caution and Recommendations to Therapists:

Position the client with the leg lower than the head end. A seated massage may be more appropriate. Excessive pressure in the abdomen should be avoided. Encourage client to avoid smoking, alcohol, bedtime snacks and spicy food.

Notes: _____

It can be treated by altering the position during sleep with the head higher than the rest of the body. Antacids are also given to reduce the acidity of the stomach contents and thus retard the erosion of the esophageal mucosa. Drugs may also be given to increase the pressure of the sphincter. Surgery is resorted to in severe cases.

===

Gastritis

Gastrointestinal system

An inflammation of the mucosa of the stomach.

Cause:

Any condition that irritates the gastric mucosa and produces inflammation causes gastritis.

Signs and Symptoms:

The person presents with pain below the sternum (epigastric pain), indigestion, loss of appetite, nausea and vomiting. In chronic cases, there may be intolerance to spicy or fatty food. Blood may be present in the vomitus.

Risk factors:

Allergy to certain food, ingestion of spicy food, alcohol, smoking, ingestion of anti-inflammatory drugs like aspirin and indomethacin, caffeine, corticosteroid therapy are some of the risk factors. Endotoxins released from bacteria can destroy the mucosa and predispose to gastritis. Acute stress eg. burns, severe infection, surgery are other risk factors.

Caution and Recommendations to Therapists:

The epigastric (upper abdominal) region may be painful to touch. Avoid the local area.

Notes: ————————————————————————————————

It is treated by alteration of diet to small frequent meals and avoidance of risk factors. Encourage client to take antacids frequently and to take drugs that may predispose to gastritis, after a meal.

German Measles (Rubella)

Integumentary, Cardiovascular systems

A viral disease that produces skin rashes.

Cause:

It is causes by the Rubella virus. It is transmitted by contact with airborne droplets of the respiratory secretion from an infected individual. The incubation period ranges from 16-18 days.

Signs and Symptoms:

The symptoms are very mild. Most often, especially in children, no fever or other systemic illness is seen. Mild skin rash is observed. The rash begins in the head and rapidly spreads downwards in a few days and soon disappears. Some individuals do not develop even a rash. Joint pain and enlargement of the occipital lymph nodes may be seen.

If it affects the fetus in a pregnant woman, it can produce congenital heart abnormalities, mental retardation, cataracts and motor and sensory nervous problems.

Risk factors:

Exposure to an infected individual increases the risk.

Caution and Recommendations to Therapists:

It is important for all female children and adults in the reproductive age group to be immunized against rubella due to the possibility of fetal abnormalities, if infected during the early stages of pregnancy.

Encourage female clients at risk to get vaccinated. Therapists should consider getting vaccinated against this disease.

Notes: ───

Gingivitis

Gastrointestinal system

An inflammation of the gums.

Cause:

It could be caused by lack of vitamins, diabetes or poor oral hygiene.

Signs and Symptoms:

It presents as redness and painless swelling of tissue around the teeth. The gum bleeds easily. It can eventually lead to loss of teeth.

Risk factors:

See cause. Poor oral hygiene can predispose to this condition.

Caution and Recommendations to Therapists:

Avoid local area if painful. Encourage client to go for regular dental checkups.

Notes: ───

Glomerulonephritis

An inflammation of the glomeruli of the kidney.

Cause:

The most common cause is the immune reaction that occurs 10-14 days after a streptococcal infection - impetigo or throat infection. The antigen-antibody complexes formed as a result of the immune system's assault on the bacteria get entrapped in the capillaries that supply the glomeruli. There is an inflammatory reaction to the complexes in the glomeruli, making the capillary membrane leaky to red cells and proteins that normally do not leave the blood vessels.

There is no cause identified for some types of glomerulonephritis.

Signs and Symptoms:

The person usually gives a history of sore throat 1-3 weeks before the onset of symptoms. There is generalized edema and fatigue. The volume of urine excreted is reduced and may be pink (presence of blood) and cloudy (presence of proteins).

Risk factors:

Untreated streptococcal infections may lead to this condition.

Caution and Recommendations to Therapists:

A very light, soothing massage of short duration is recommended. Do not try to reduce the edema present as the cause is not inadequate drainage of interstitial fluid. Rather, the edema actually prevents overloading of the heart which is overly stressed by the accumulation of fluid.

Notes:

Treatment is mainly supportive, with maintenance of fluid and electrolyte balance and diet restrictions - reduced water, protein and salt intake.

Glomerulonephritis can progress to nephrotic syndrome and kidney failure.

Glossitis

An inflammation of the tongue.

Cause:

The inflammation may be due to Streptococcal infection, irritation or injury to the tongue, hypersensitivity or vitamin deficiency.

Signs and Symptoms:

The tongue is red and swollen and may be ulcerated. There is pain on swallowing and chewing. The swelling of the tongue along with the pain can make speech difficult.

Risk factors:

Irregular biting surface of teeth, ill-fitting dentures, injury to tongue caused during convulsions, spicy food, alcohol, smoking, allergy to toothpaste and vitamin deficiency are all predisposing factors.

Caution and Recommendations to Therapists:

If the glossitis is due to hypersensitivity, it is possible for the client to be allergic to aroma therapy, or to oils that are used during massage. Obtain a thorough history and avoid use of allergic substances.

Notes: ─────────────────────────────────────

Treatment of underlying cause, good oral hygiene, mouth washes and avoidance of predisposing factors are the treatment options used.

Goiter (Simple goiter, Nontoxic goiter)   Endocrine system

An enlargement of the thyroid gland.

Cause:

It usually results when the production of thyroid hormone does not meet the metabolic needs. It may be due to lack of adequate iodine in the diet. Such a condition may be seen in communities living in areas with iodine-depleted soil. When the demands are more for the hormone as during pregnancy, adolescence and menopause, the thyroid gland may hypertrophy especially if the iodine needs are not met. Certain foods have a direct effect on thyroxine production. Intake of excess rutabagas, cabbage, soybeans, peanuts, peaches, peas, strawberries, spinach and radishes can reduce thyroxine production.

Signs and Symptoms:

The thyroid enlarges in size slowly and presents as a painless, uniform or nodular swelling in front of the neck. The swelling moves on swallowing. Usually there are no signs of hyper or hypothyroidism - but may present as either. Due to the compression of the underlying structures, the person may have difficulty in swallowing. Pressure on the neck veins can cause the veins above the swelling to bulge and become prominent.

Risk factors:

See Cause.

Caution and Recommendations to Therapists:

Encourage client to consult a physician if a thyroid swelling is noted as the cause has to be found and tumors have to be ruled out. Do not massage over the neck area.

Notes: ──

The thyroid gland is located in front of the neck and weighs about 30 grams. It is butterfly shaped with two lobes on either side of the trachea. The lobes are about 5cm long, 2cm thick and about 3cm wide. A normal thyroid is not visible and is felt as a soft mass in front of the neck above the sternum, that moves up on swallowing.

Gonorrhea

Reproductive system

A sexually transmitted disease caused by bacteria.

Cause:

It is caused by the bacteria Neisseria gonorrhoeae which can survive only for a very short duration outside the human body. It is transmitted through intimate physical contact. Infection can also spread from an infected mother to the baby during delivery. The bacteria enters the mucosal membrane producing inflammation. The bacteria can change its form easily and evade local immune reaction. Hence repeated infections are possible in an individual.

Signs and Symptoms:

In men it presents as inflammation of the urethra 1-8 days after infection. Pain on urination and profuse white discharge is common. The infection may travel upwards and produce inflammation of the epididymis, prostate and other areas.

In women, pain on urination, profuse white discharge, increased and abnormal menstrual bleeding are common. The infection may spread upwards and cause inflammation of the fallopian tubes and other areas. The resolution of the inflammation by fibrosis can produce narrowing of the tubes and increase the chances of infertility and ectopic pregnancy. There may be lower abdominal pain and pain during intercourse.

Risk factors:

It is common in the lower socioeconomic group in urban areas. Those with a past history of gonorrhea are at higher risk. The incidence is highest in the sexually active adolescent female.

Caution and Recommendations to Therapists:

Refer client to physician if they give a history of white discharge and pain on passing urine. Since the infection spreads by intimate physical contact - specifically sexual intercourse, and does not live for very long outside the human body the risk of the therapist contracting the infection is very low.

Notes:

The disease is easily treated with antibiotics.

Guillain-Barre Syndrome (Infectious polyneuritis, Landry - Guillain - Barre syndrome, Acute idiopathic polyneuritis)
Nervous system

An acute, rapidly progressive disorder that results in muscle weakness and sensory loss.

Cause:

The cause is unknown. But it may be due to the alteration of the body's immunity to attack antigens in peripheral nerves. This seems to follow many forms of viral infections including AIDS and Hepatitis. There is inflammation and swelling around peripheral nerves with destruction of myelin sheath, sensory and motor neurons.

Signs and Symptoms:

There is usually a history of mild fever or respiratory infection preceding the disease. Muscle weakness of legs, followed by weakness of the arms and face are seen. The signs and symptoms appear over a few days. The weakness may be accompanied by pain and stiffness. There may be loss of sensation. Weakness of the respiratory muscles can result in death.

Autonomic disturbances may also be seen. This presents as postural hypotension, abnormal sweating, flushing of face, bladder and bowel disorders. Typically, the syndrome has three phases - the initial phase lasting for 1-3 weeks when the symptoms are seen, the plateau phase lasting for about 2 weeks when the symptoms do not progress and the recovery phase which may last from months to years. Recovery may not be complete. The debility makes the person prone to infections. Muscle contractures, joint stiffness, deep vein thrombosis (following prolonged immobility) are other complications.

Risk factors:

Surgery, influenza vaccination, viral illness, Hodgkin's disease and Lupus Erythematosus may precipitate the disease.

Caution and Recommendations to Therapists:

During the active and plateau phase, massage helps improve circulation and reduce pain. Perform passive range of motion exercises within the pain tolerance. Movement of shoulder, thighs and trunk muscles are painful in these individuals. Use tapotement and vibration strokes over the chest to help mucus drainage from the lungs. Since these individuals are in bed they are prone for pressure ulcers. Gently massage areas that are prone for ulcers - these areas are around the sacrum, ankles and heels. Avoid massaging a wide area around the ulcer if an ulcer has already developed. Sensory loss in certain areas of the body will result in the client giving inadequate feedback. Avoid using excessive pressure.

Individuals with this disorder are prone to postural hypotension. Support the client well when changing positions. They are also prone to thrombophlebitis (inflammation of veins) especially in the legs. Watch for edema, pain, redness and swelling in the legs. Do not massage the legs if this is present as you may dislodge a thrombus and produce further complications. If the client has constipation give a stimulatory abdominal massage (always in a clockwise direction).

In the recovery phase the aim is to prevent contractures and increase tone of the flaccid muscles. Use stimulatory massage over flaccid muscles. Perform passive range of motion exercises of all joints. Use deep transverse friction around joints to reduce adhesions and stretch tendons. Avoid excessive pressure over areas with sensory loss. If the client is in a wheelchair, spend time massaging muscles that are stressed excessively while maneuvering the wheelchair.

Notes: _____

Guillain-Barre Syndrome is treated initially with steroids to reduce inflammation. Supportive measures are taken to maintain vital functions and prevent complications. Although a viral infection is implicated, it is not infectious.

Hay Fever (Allergic rhinitis)   Respiratory system

An inflammation of the nose and conjunctiva that occurs seasonally due to allergy.

Cause:

Individuals who are genetically predisposed, react to certain antigens like pollen, fungal spores, by producing large amounts of immunoglobulins (antibodies). The antigen antibody reaction is responsible for the symptoms seen..

Signs and Symptoms:

Recurrent sneezing, watery nasal discharge, itching (pruritus), congestion and swelling of the eyes and nose, itching in the throat and headache are the most common symptoms.

Risk factors:

Hay fever can occur in all age groups, but is more common in children and adolescents. A genetic predisposition is also present.

Caution and Recommendations for Therapists:

Individuals with allergic rhinitis may also have other forms of allergy, so a proper and detailed history of allergy should be taken. Keep the clinic area dust free to prevent a fresh episode of rhinitis in these individuals. Proper air conditioning, regular vacuuming, low humidity, avoiding use of dust-collecting items like thick carpets and heavy drapes, minimizing presence or avoidance of flowering plants are some of the simple precautions that can be taken in the clinic to reduce the incidence of allergy in clients. Refer client to local support groups for Allergy. See Appendix IV for resources.

Notes: _____

Headache - cluster

Headaches of short duration occurring recurrently for short periods of time.

Cause:

The cause is not known. They are considered to be a vascular type of headache.

Signs and Symptoms:

The headache lasts from 10 minutes to two hours. The pain is confined to the eye and nose of one side causing watering of the eye and running of the nose. There may be redness of the skin on the side of pain. The headache recurs 2-3 times a day for 5-6 weeks. There may be no headaches for weeks to months after the cluster of symptoms.

Risk factors:

It may be induced by stress.

Caution and Recommendations to Therapists:

It is usually not treated as it lasts only for a short while. During an attack the same techniques as for tension headache may be used (see Headache -Tension) .

Notes:

Vasoconstrictors or inhalation of pure oxygen is used to treat this type of headache.

Headache - migraine

A throbbing pain in the head that is often confined to one side of the head, associated with or without an aura.

Cause:

The cause is unknown. Recent evidence indicates that the headache is brought on by the leakiness of the blood vessels of the brain due to polypeptides called neurokinin that dilate blood vessels. Abnormal metabolism and decrease of serotonin (5 hydroxy tryptamine) in the brain have also been implicated. Migraine has been associated with dilatation and constriction of arteries inside and outside the cranium.

Signs and Symptoms:

The pain is usually confined to one side of the head initially, later spreading to other areas. The head ache is typically preceded by flashing lights, dark spots, double vision and hallucinations. These auras are due to the reduced blood flow to specific areas of the brain. Nausea, vomiting, hypersensitivity to light, sound and smell are other typical symptoms. Migraine can also occur without auras.

Risk factors:

Different factors precipitate an attack in susceptible individuals. Red wine, cheese, canned food, hot dog, salami, bacon - food containing preservatives, bean pods, chocolate, avocados, bananas, citrus fruits, yogurt, sour cream, fresh bread, coffee cake, doughnuts, nuts, peanut butter, fermented, pickled and marinated foods are some of the food types that may precipitate an attack. In some, changes in weather and pressure can cause a headache. In women, the hormonal changes during the menstrual cycle can also trigger an attack. In the younger age group both males and females are equally affected. In adults, women are attacked more than men. There may be a family history of migraine headache.

Caution and Recommendations to Therapists:

During the headache, a whole body relaxation massage is most helpful. Use same techniques as for tension headache when massaging over the neck, scalp and face. Do not apply heat over the area as it causes changes in the arteries that may increase the pain. During the headache apply cold compresses or gel packs to the face, scalp, eyes, wrist and feet. Use deep moist heat at the end of treatment.

The treatment regimen followed is once a week for one month followed by once every other week for a total of eight weeks. Thirty minute sessions have been found to be adequate. Other recommended treatment schedules are a total of 10-12 sessions lasting about 15 minutes each scheduled every other day.

Consider keeping brochures of local migraine associations in the clinic. Encourage client to make dietary and life-style changes. Advice client to do aerobic exercises regularly. This promotes circulation. Teach clients to massage the scalp and neck muscles. Refer clients to local groups (see Appendix IV).

Notes:

Cranio sacral training is one form of treatment. Deep breathing exercises and imagery have been found to be effective by some.

Headache - others

Includes headaches that are not tension or migraine.

Cause:

Headaches can be caused by infection of the meninges - meningitis, tumors that increase the intracranial tension, disorders of the cranium, neck, eyes, ears, nose, sinuses, teeth, mouth or other facial/cranial structures. Pressure, reduced blood supply or inflammation of the main sensory nerve - the trigeminal nerve can also cause severe pain (see trigeminal neuralgia). Headaches may also be caused by withdrawal syndrome associated with alcohol or substance abuse. The pain may be referred from temporomandibular joint syndrome or problems with the cervical spine.

Signs and Symptoms:

Headaches due to meningitis, or other intracranial problems are often associated with motor or sensory problems. There will also be neck stiffness and pain on flexing the hip with the knee extended. The pain is produced by the stretching of the inflamed meninges when performing this maneuver. Those caused by tumors are typically associated with nausea and forceful vomiting. The client will also give a history of recent onset of headache.

Risk factors:

See Causes

Caution and Recommendations to Therapists:

It is very important to take a careful and detailed history when dealing with headache. Refer to physician if the history indicates any of the above lesions. Massage is indicated only for tension or migraine headaches.

Notes:

Although the pain fibres from other parts of the body reach the brain which interprets it, the brain by itself does not have pain fibres!

Headache - tension (Fibrositic)

Nervous, Musculoskeletal systems

A symptom of pain in the head, face and/or neck regions due to muscle contraction and psychological causes.

Cause:

This is the commonest type of headache. Contraction/spasm of the neck and scalp muscles caused by stress of any kind produce this type of headache. The pain is produced by the pressure of the contracted muscle on the nerves and blood vessels in the area. The resultant reduced blood flow increases the accumulation of waste products like lactic acid in the area which perpetuate the pain.

Signs and Symptoms:

The client complains of a dull, persistent ache and a feeling of tightness around the head, temple, forehead and occiput. The pain is typically more in the evenings. There is no loss of sensation, muscle weakness, or aura associated with this type. Headaches that start suddenly in a person who has not experienced such headache before is not tension headache.

Risk factors:

Noise, bright lights, crowds, mental strain, menstruation, alcohol intake, fasting and fatigue can precipitate an attack. Any occupation which requires the head to be held in a fixed position such as typing, jewellery repair or microscope work can increase the risk of contracting this type of headache. Prolonged exposure to cold, sleeping with held in a strained position also predispose to this condition.

Caution and Recommendations to Therapists:

Encourage client to sleep in a warm room and tie a scarf around the neck if venturing out in the cold. Take a good history and try to identify the precipitating cause of the headache. Massage can help only temporarily, but identifying and avoiding precipitating factors alone can produce long-term effects.

Ask client to actively contract the shoulder and neck muscles and then relax it as much as possible. This helps the client to consciously relax muscles that are being involuntarily tensed. Position the client in a seated position with the head resting on a pillow in front, supported by elevated arms. This helps to relax the shoulder and neck muscles. The aim is to relax the muscles in spasm and thereby relieve the pressure on the nerves and blood vessels. The aim is also to promote venous and lymphatic drainage from the area. Moist heat application over the tense muscles during the treatment have been found to be beneficial. Use effleurage, friction and vibration strokes in the shoulder and neck region. Effleurage should be long and continuous beginning from the occiput to the shoulder joint and from below, over the scapula to the neck - ie. in the direction of the muscle fibres of the trapezius.

Friction is done on either side of the spinous process of the cervical vertebrae. Start friction in areas that are less tense and then slowly progress to that under spasm. Use the pads of your fingers and start with lighter strokes and then proceed to deeper strokes. Make the strokes continuous ie. do friction from one area to the adjacent area without loosing contact with the skin. Alternate the friction strokes with effleurage from time to time.

Do not neglect to massage the neck muscles - scalene and sternocleidomastoid which are in front of the neck. More time should be spent over the origin and the insertion of these muscles which will be closer to the clavicle and sternum and the mastoid process (the protrusion just behind the ear) respectively. The massage should also focuss on the trapezius, erector spinae, levator scapulae and rhomboids muscles that are usually tense. Use vibration over the trigger point areas for five to ten seconds, repeating the vibration after eight to ten seconds while maintaining contact with the skin during the break. Repeat the procedure three to four times.

Passively move the head and neck in all directions. Gentle traction of the head also helps. Initially, spend half the duration of massage using effleurage with the rest of the time divided equally for vibration and friction strokes. Increase the duration spent on friction in subsequent sessions up to three fourth of the time. Gentle scalp and face massage have also been found to be very beneficial. Spend time over the temporalis (the fan shaped muscle located above the ears), masseters and frontalis (located in the forehead region) using finger tip kneading strokes.

Four to five sessions for the first week followed by less frequent sessions for a total of twelve treatment sessions have been found to be beneficial. The duration of each session should be short not lasting for more than 15 minutes. Other treatment schedules practised are two times a week for two weeks followed by once a week for one month. Individualize the treatment according to the client's feedback. There may be a need to charge the client on a treatment schedule basis rather than individual sessions.

The client may be on pain killers and therefore give inadequate feedback. Adjust pressures accordingly.

Notes: _____

Numerous conditions can precipitate a headache and treatment varies according to cause. A proper history and identification of the cause is very important. Imagery, biofeedback are other techniques employed to combat headache. A 2% dilution of lavender and peppermint (essential oil) in a carrier oil has also been used by some. Such a dilution can be obtained by mixing 20 drops of the essential oil to 50 ml. of carrier oil.

Heart attack (Myocardial Infarction)

Cardiovascular system

Death of myocardial tissue due to insufficient blood flow in the coronary arteries.

Cause:

Insufficient coronary blood flow due to thrombosis, vasospasm, or increased oxygen demand by the myocardium causes this condition..

Signs and Symptoms:

The person presents with an abrupt onset of suffocating, squeezing or crushing pain below the sternum, or radiating to the left arm, jaw or neck. The pain is not relieved by rest or drugs for angina. It may be associated with nausea and vomiting or indigestion. The pain may be accompanied by palpitations, restlessness and anxiety. The skin may be pale and moist. Complications include sudden death, shock, rupture of the heart, thromboemboli, ventricular aneurysms and pericarditis.

Risk factors:

Atherosclerosis predisposes to myocardial infarction. See risk factors for atherosclerosis and angina.

Caution and Recommendations to Therapists:

Avoid using stimulatory or painful techniques in clients with atherosclerosis, angina or previous myocardial infarction. A whole body, gentle relaxation massage alleviates stress, a common precipitator of heart attack.

Notes: _____

Heart Failure

Cardiovascular system

A syndrome where the heart is unable to cope with the demands made by the body.

Cause:

Heart failure may be due to many conditions. The dysfunction may be due to damage to the heart muscle as in coronary artery disease and myocardial infarction. It may be due to mechanical disturbances as in stenosis (narrowing) of the opening between the ventricle and atrium, rapid beating of the heart as in atrial fibrillation can lead to inefficiency in pumping the blood from the heart. Heart failure can also occur when the heart is overloaded by increased pressure in the blood vessels (hypertension; aortic stenosis) or leaky valves.

To compensate for the reduced blood that is pumped, the heart increases in size by dilation and/or hypertrophy. Another compensatory mechanism is the increase in heart rate due to increased sympathetic activity.

Signs and Symptoms:

The signs and symptoms produced by heart failure depends on whether the right side, the left side or both sides of the heart fail. If the right ventricle is affected, there is a tendency for the blood to dam up in the venous circulation. This results in edema of the legs, sacral region and enlargement of the liver and spleen. Fluid may collect in the abdomen (ascites).

In left heart failure, pressure tends to build up in the pulmonary circulation causing pulmonary edema and difficulty in and noisy breathing.

The inadequate blood flow to the brain and kidney can produce other symptoms.

Risk factors:

See Cause.

Caution and Recommendations to Therapists:

It is important to find out the cause of edema in any edematous client. If cardiac edema is suspected, refer to a physician.

Techniques to reduce edema are not beneficial, and in fact may be detrimental in a client in cardiac failure.

Notes:

The underlying pathology has to be identified for proper treatment. Diuretics, low salt intake are some of the other supportive measures used.

Hemophilia
Cardiovascular system

A hereditary bleeding disorder due to deficiency of a specific clotting factor in the blood.

Cause:

Hemophilia A, one of the types, is caused by a lack of Factor VIII, which is one of the clotting factors. Lack of factor IX is said to be responsible for Hemophilia B.

The clotting mechanism is complex and requires the activation of many inactive factors present in the blood. Absence of any of these factors can result in dysfunction of the clotting mechanism. Hemophilia is inherited from the mother - ie. the gene responsible for the deficiency is present in the X chromosome. Since it is recessive, it does not present in the daughter if the other X chromosome is normal. However, the daughter can be a carrier of the gene and transmit it to the son. Since there is only one X chromosome in males, presence of the gene results in presentation of the disease in the form of bleeding.

Signs and Symptoms:

Depending on the degree of deficiency, the person presents with mild, moderate or severe forms of abnormal bleeding. In the mild form, prolonged bleeding may be seen only after major trauma. In the severe form the person may bleed spontaneously. Large hematomas may form in the muscle or under the skin with the mildest of trauma. Bleeding into the joints can lead to severe pain, swelling and joint stiffness that is permanent. Internal bleeding can lead to shock and death.

Risk factors:

A family history of the disease increases the risk.

Caution and Recommendations to Therapists:

Suspect a bleeding disorder in a client with large hematomas. Elevation of the limb and cold compresses may be of benefit to slow the bleeding process. Massage is contraindicated in those with severe forms of hemophilia. In the milder forms, very superficial, light strokes may not produce harm to the client. In any event, it is advisable to consult the Physician before any form of massage is under taken.

Refer client to a local support group. Encourage daughters born into families with a history of hemophilia to have genetic counseling. Refer to Appendix IV for resources.

Notes: ─────────────────────────────────────

Since these individuals require frequent transfusions, there is a risk of human Immunodeficiency Virus infection through blood products.

Hemorrhoids
Gastrointestinal, Cardiovascular systems

A condition with abnormal dilatation of veins in the rectum.

Cause:

It is caused by increased pressure in the venous network of the rectum.

Signs and Symptoms:

Hemorrhoids usually present with no symptoms or as passage of fresh blood during defecation. If the hemorrhoids are chronic, they may be seen or felt as soft swellings in the anus. Itching around the anus is often present. If the hemorrhoid gets obstructed, a sharp pain may be experienced in the anal area. Chronic bleeding through the anus can result in anemia in the client.

Risk factors:

Occupations that involve prolonged standing or sitting; chronic constipation or diarrhea where straining occurs; chronic cough which recurrently increase the intra-abdominal pressure; any condition that results in damming up of blood in the veins such as cirrhosis of the liver and heart failure are all predisposing factors. Conditions that weaken the pelvic floor - old age, rectal surgery, pregnancy and episiotomy (an incision that is made in the pelvic floor to widen the outlet for the baby during labor) also increase the risk of hemorrhoids.

Caution and Recommendations to Therapists:

Encourage client to alter diet and avoid prolonged standing, sitting and straining. Obtain a good history to determine the cause of hemorrhoids. Massage is not contraindicated, but avoid excessive pressure in the abdominal area.

Notes:

It is treated with pain killers. Measures to reduce the pressure include regulation of bowel habits, alteration of diet to include raw vegetables, fruits and whole grain cereal. The pain can be reduced by local anaesthetic creams and sitting in a warm water bath. Injection of sclerosing agents or surgery are strategies used for severe cases.

Hepatitis   Gastrointestinal system

An inflammation of the liver

Cause:

There are many factors that can cause this condition, a few of which are infectious.

Inflammation of the liver can be caused by alcohol, drugs and toxins. Malaria (a parasitic infection), infectious mononucleosis, typhoid, amebiasis are infectious causes of hepatitis. More commonly, hepatitis is due to infection by the hepatitis virus. The hepatitis virus exists as many strains. Hepatitis A, B, B associated delta, C and E viruses are some of the well known strains. The mode of transmission and incubation period vary from strain to strain.

Hepatitis A infection, also known as infectious hepatitis or short incubation hepatitis is highly contagious and is transmitted by the fecal-oral route. It is transmitted by ingestion of contaminated food, water or milk. Commonly, it is spread by eating shell fish from infected water. In homosexuals it can spread by oral-anal contact. It is rarely transmitted through intravenous blood or plasma as the virus is present in the blood during symptoms - a period when the client is unlikely to donate. The incubation period is 15-45 days. In the infected person the virus can be seen in the feces even two weeks before the onset of symptoms and persists in the feces for many weeks after symptoms begin.

Hepatitis B infection, also known as serum hepatitis is more serious than Hepatitis A. It lasts longer and can lead to cirrhosis, cancer of the liver and a carrier state. Carrier state is the state of a person when the virus continues to be excreted even though no symptoms are seen. It has a long incubation period of 1.5 to 2 months. The symptoms may last from weeks to months. The virus is usually transmitted through infected blood, serum or plasma. However, it can spread by oral or sexual contact as it is present in most body secretions. Infants can contract it from infected mothers. Infected individuals can be carriers for months and years ie. they are capable of transmitting the disease during this period.

Hepatitis C is known as non-A, non-B hepatitis and can cause acute or chronic hepatitis. This can also lead to a carrier state and liver cancer. It is transmitted through blood transfusions or exposure to blood products.

Hepatitis D virus infection or B associated delta virus, affects individuals who are infected by the B virus. It makes the symptoms associated with Hepatitis B infection more severe. Carrier states are also seen. It is prevented by taking preventive measures against Hepatitis B infection.

Hepatitis E is transmitted by the fecal-oral route and the symptoms are short lived, similar to that of Hepatitis A.

Signs and Symptoms:

The symptoms are a result of the direct liver cell injury by the virus as well as the immune response of the body to the infection. The symptoms vary from no symptoms to severe jaundice, liver failure and death. In the early stages, the person experiences muscle and joint pain, easy fatiguability, loss of appetite, nausea, vomiting, diarrhea or constipation. Dull pain in the right upper abdomen may be present. Slowly this leads to jaundice, liver and spleen enlargement. The acute illness usually lasts for 2-3 weeks. The recovery of the person depends on the type of hepatitis. A person with Hepatitis A recovers in about 9 weeks while an individual with Hepatitis B and C takes about 16 weeks.

Risk factors:

The incidence is higher in intravenous drug abusers, those requiring blood products (people with bleeding disorders), homosexuals and heterosexuals. Health care workers exposed to blood products or high risk individuals, infants born to infected mothers, AIDS victims, hemodialysis patients and individuals on immunosuppressants are all at risk.

Caution and Recommendations to Therapists:

Always contact physician about the infectivity of an individual with history of hepatitis. Hepatitis as a side effect of drugs or alcohol intake is not infective. Hepatitis A, B ,C, D and E are all infective with potential for the person to be in a carrier state. It is advisable to massage individuals with history of this condition with the underclothes on. Take special precautions to wash hands thoroughly with soap and disinfect the linen. Avoid massage to abdomen (especially the right upper quadrant) if there is a history of chronic Hepatitis (hepatitis lasting for more than 6 months).

It is advisable for all therapists to be vaccinated against hepatitis B. Three doses are given at 0, 1 and 6 months.

Notes: ────────────────────────────────────

Immunoglobulin (antibodies) against Hepatitis A can be given to people in close contact with an infected person, or to those travelling to areas (India, Africa, Asia or Central America) where hepatitis A is endemic. The immunity is short lived and booster doses are required.

Vaccines are available for Hepatitis B in the form of Hepatitis B immunoglobulin (antibodies). This provides protection for 3-6 months. Another form of Hepatitis B vaccine provides long term immunity. The latter is recommended for people in occupations at high risk. This includes massage therapists.

Hepatitis is treated symptomatically, with bedrest, regulation of fat intake and avoidance of alcohol and drugs that are toxic to the liver.

Hernia - femoral

A protrusion of an organ lying inside the abdominal cavity, through an abnormal opening around the femoral artery as it goes into the leg in the groin area.

Cause:

Weakness of the muscles and fascia of the abdomen along with increased intra abdominal pressure results in the intestines, omentum or bladder to protrude through this potential weak spot called the femoral canal.

Signs and Symptoms:

It presents as a swelling that is soft and reducible located just below the crease in the upper part of the thigh. Rarely, it can cause severe pain with nausea and vomiting, if a part of the intestines get obstructed.

Risk factors:

Straining, lifting weights, or chronic persistent cough can predispose to this.

Caution and Recommendations to Therapists:

Advice the client to consult a physician if a painless reducible or irreducible swelling is seen. Do not massage over the hernia or try to reduce the swelling as obstruction or perforation can be produced in the bowel. Encourage client to reduce weight and get treated for cough if present. Advice the client to avoid lifting and straining. A normal relaxation massage to other parts of the body is beneficial.

Notes:

Hernia is treated with a truss to support and reduce the swelling if in an elderly individual or in those who cannot have surgery. Surgically, steel mesh, wires or fascia can be used to reinforce the weakened area and or the opening closed after the contents are pushed into the abdomen.

Hernia - hiatal (Hiatus hernia)　　Gastrointestinal system

An abnormal opening in the diaphragm that allows a portion of the stomach to enter the thoracic cavity.

Cause:

It is commonly caused by weakening of the diaphragmatic muscle. Other conditions that increase the intra-abdominal pressure also cause this.

Signs and Symptoms:

Usually it does not produce any symptoms. If it is associated with esophageal reflux, there is burning pain below the sternum especially a few hours after a meal. If part of the stomach is caught in the opening such that the blood flow is compromised, there is severe pain and the person may go into shock.

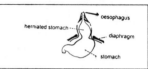

Risk factors:

It is more common in the older age group. The incidence is higher in women. Kyphoscoliosis, trauma, obesity, pregnancy, extreme physical exertion, tight clothings that tend to constrict the abdomen, chronic coughs and straining predispose to this condition.

Caution and Recommendations to Therapists:

Massage should be given in a seated position if the individual is uncomfortable supine or prone.

Notes:

It is managed conservatively by avoiding activities that increase the intra abdominal pressure. Drugs may be given to improve the pressure of the esophageal sphincter. Diet is also modified by encouraging the individual to eat small quantities at a time, but increasing the frequency. Antacids are given to reduce the acidity. Surgery is another treatment option.

Hernia - incisional

Musculoskeletal, Gastrointestinal systems

Protrusion of an organ lying inside the abdominal cavity, through an incision site of a previous surgery.

Cause:

This occurs usually if the incision site on the abdominal wall is weak.

Signs and Symptoms:

It presents as a painless, reducible or irreducible swelling in and around the incisional site. Movements of the intestines can be seen if the swelling is produced by intestines. The swelling becomes more prominent on coughing or straining and may reduce on lying down. Severe, pain, nausea and vomiting is produced if the intestines are obstructed or twisted and emergency surgery is required.

Risk factors:

Infection of the incision site, or delayed wound healing increase the risk. Straining, lifting weights, or chronic persistent cough before proper healing of the wound can also predispose to this.

Caution and Recommendations to Therapists:

see Hernia - femoral.

Notes: _____

see Hernia - femoral.

===

Hernia - inguinal

Musculoskeletal, Gastrointestinal systems

The protrusion of an organ lying inside the abdominal cavity, through an abnormal opening in the inguinal (upper part of the groin) region.

Cause:

Weakness of the muscles and fascia of the abdomen along with increased intra abdominal pressure results in the intestines, omentum or bladder to protrude through this potential weak spot. In males, the testis descends from the abdomen into the scrotum through the inguinal canal during the seventh month of gestation. If this inguinal canal does not close properly, the organs from the abdomen can be forced into the canal to appear as a swelling in the groin area. Inguinal hernias can also occur in females as the round ligament (a ligament that supports the uterus) passes through this canal.

Signs and Symptoms:

It usually presents as a painless swelling that becomes more prominent on straining. Sometimes if the intestine has herniated, peristalsis (movement of the intestines) can be seen. Most hernias are reducible and can be pushed back manually or reduce on lying down. If adhesions are present between the organ and the surrounding tissue, the hernia cannot be reduced. If the protruding part of the intestines become blocked or twisted, there is severe pain over the area along with nausea and vomiting. In such cases, emergency surgery has to be performed.

Risk factors:

Weakness of the abdominal wall with aging, obesity and pregnancy predispose to this condition. Occupations which involve heavy lifting and straining increase the intraabdominal pressure. Chronic constipation, chronic cough are other predisposing factors. Birth malformations and nonclosure of the inguinal canal can also be a risk factor.

Caution and Recommendations to Therapists:

See Hernia - femoral.

Notes: ───

See Hernia - femoral.

Hernia - umbilical

Musculoskeletal, Gastrointestinal systems

Protrusion of an organ lying inside the abdominal cavity, through an abnormal opening around the umbilicus (belly button/navel).

Cause:

Weakness of the muscles and fascia of the abdomen along with increased intra abdominal pressure results in the intestines, omentum or bladder to protrude through this potential weak spot.

Signs and Symptoms:

It presents as a painless, reducible or irreducible swelling around the umbilicus. Movements of the intestines can be seen if the swelling is produced by intestines. The swelling becomes more prominent on coughing or straining and may reduce on lying down. Severe, pain, nausea and vomiting is produced if the intestines are obstructed or twisted and emergency surgery is required.

Risk factors:

In the newborn, weak or abnormal muscle structures around the umbilical cord can result in an umbilical hernia which disappears before the age of five. Obese individuals, or those who have had multiple pregnancies are also prone. This hernia is also seen in those in occupations which involve lifting and straining or in those with chronic constipation or cough.

Caution and Recommendations to Therapists:

See Hernia - femoral.

Notes:

See Hernia - femoral.

Herpes Simplex (Cold sore, Fever blister)

Integumentary system

A viral infection of the skin and mucous membrane.

Cause:

It is caused by Herpes simplex virus Type I and type II. Infections of the genitalia are caused by Type I and II while those above the waist are caused by Type I. It is spread by direct, intimate contact, oral sex and kissing, when the virus is inoculated into the small cracks in the skin or mucous membrane. The virus may produce symptoms straight away (primary herpes) or migrate to the ganglia of sensory nerve where it may lie dormant and later get reactivated (secondary herpes). The incubation period for primary herpes is 5-14 days.

Signs and Symptoms:

In the primary type the client presents with high fever, sore throat and vesicles all over the mucous membrane. In the general form, pain, itching, vaginal discharge and painful enlargement of the lymph node may be present. The virus may be shed from the lesions upto 12 days after the symptoms are seen. The virus persists in the ganglia and are reactivated in some people. This is secondary herpes. The client complains of burning and itching sensations in the affected area. Soon the area reddens with formation of vesicles that progress to pustules, ulcer and crusts. There may be accompanying pain. The lesion disappears in 10-14 days. It commonly affects the face, mouth or lips.

Risk factors:

Previous infection by herpes virus is a risk factor. There is a recurrence of infection precipitated by stress, exposure to sunlight, menstruation or injury.

Caution and Recommendations to Therapists:

It is infectious in an active state so avoid massage. Herpes can be spread from one part of the body to another by direct contact and is an occupational hazard for therapists.

Notes: _____

Once infected, a high incidence of recurrence is seen.

Herpes Zoster (Shingles)

Integumentary, Nervous systems

A viral infection of spinal or cranial nerves, affecting a dermatome segment of the skin.

Cause:

It is caused by the herpes virus that causes chickenpox. The virus, which may lie latent in the dorsal root ganglion of a nerve for years in a person who has been exposed to chicken pox, is reactivated and travels along the dermatome causing an inflammatory reaction.

Signs and Symptoms:

Vesicles with reddened bases erupt unilaterally, confined to a single or adjacent group of dermatomes, over a period of 3-4 days. It may be preceded by fever,

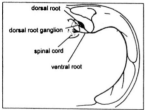

itching, pain and tenderness in the area. The vesicles dry and form crusts over a period of 2-3weeks. If the branch of the trigeminal nerve supplying the eye is involved it may result in blindness. Older clients may experience prolonged pain in the area even in the absence of vesicles. The severity varies from person to person. Pain may vary from mild to excruciating and may be permanent pain. (see Appendix 1 figure:5)

Risk factors:

Immunocompromised individuals and those highly stressed are more prone.

Caution and Recommendations to Therapists:

It is contagious when the vesicles erupt. Contact with the virus results in chicken pox in a person who has never been exposed to it. Avoid massage during the acute phase. Massage may be given during the intermittent phases when there is no visible lesion, and is beneficial to the client. No specific precautions need be taken when there are no vesicles. Often, elderly clients may be on pain killers if experiencing neuralgia. Always enquire about the use of pain killers before massage. Excessive pressure during massage can damage skin and tissue in clients with reduced sensitivity to pain sensations.

Notes: _____

Hodgkin's disease (Lymphoma - Hodgekin's)

Lymphatic system

A malignant disorder of the lymphatic structures.

Cause:

The cause is not known. It is suspected that it starts as an inflammatory reaction to an infectious agent in an individual whose immunity is lowered or deficient.

Signs and Symptoms:

It presents as a painless, progressive enlargement of a single or group of lymph nodes with a potential to spread to other areas. Fever, night sweats, unexplained weight loss, fatigue, itching and anemia are some of the symptoms. In advanced stages, due to the effect of the abnormal lymphocytes of the immune system, the immunity is lowered and the client becomes more susceptible to infections.

Risk factors:

It is more common in young adults between 15 and 35 years of age.

Caution and Recommendations to Therapists:

The disease is not contagious. However, massage is contraindicated as Hodgkin's disease is a form of cancer and massage can help spread it. Consult physician if the client is under treatment. Both the disease and treatment reduce the activity of the immune system and there is danger of exposure to mild infections having serious consequences.

Notes: _____

It is treated with radiation or chemotherapy according to the extent of the disease.

Huntington's disease (Huntington's chorea, hereditary chorea, Chronic progressive chorea, Adult chorea)

(Greek: chorea - to dance)   **Nervous system**

A degenerative disease of the cerebral cortex and basal ganglia.

Cause:

The cause is unknown but it is transmitted genetically. Both sexes can inherit it. There is a 50% chance of a child getting it from a parent who has the disease. If the child does not inherit it there is no chance of it being transmitted down the generation.It may be due to destruction of neurons that produce a neurotransmitter GABA (gama amino butyric acid) that inhibits activity in the basal ganglia.

Signs and Symptoms:

The symptoms start slowly with loss of motor control. It then progresses to rapid, involuntary, purposeless movements. The movements are often graceful hence the name chorea. The movements are confined to one side of the face, tongue or arm and then progresses to other areas. The disease then progresses to personality changes like carelessness, moodiness, inappropriate behavior, loss of memory and lack of concentration.

Risk factors:

It usually affects people between the ages of 25-55. There is a family history of the disease.

Caution and Recommendations to Therapists:

Consult physician. Refer clients to local support groups (see Appendix IV)

Notes: _____

This disease often requires institutionalization of the person. It progresses to death within 15 years of onset. Treatment is only supportive.

Hydrocephalus

An excessive accumulation of cerebrospinal fluid (CSF) within the ventricles of the brain.

Cause:

Any condition that results in obstruction to the flow of CSF from the ventricles of the brain into the venous sinuses or reduces absorption or results in overproduction of CSF can cause hydrocephalus. This usually occurs in children, but can occur in adults too. The increased pressure on the brain tissue results in atrophy and resultant mental retardation, motor function abnormalities and loss of vision.

Signs and Symptoms:

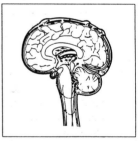

In infants the head appears abnormally large. This is due to the increased pressure separating the unfused sutures of the bones of the skull. The skin is thin and shiny and the neck muscles are weak. If the pressure is very high it can depress the orbits of the eye and the eyes look small and sunken. Motor dysfunction - spasticity of the lower legs may also occur. In adults, there may be slowing of the intellect, irritability, reduced consciousness, headache, forceful vomiting, seizures, incoordination and difficulty in maintaining balance. Since the sutures are fused in adults, there is no increase in the size of the head.

Risk factors:

Obstruction to flow can occur as a complication of meningitis, syphilis, brain tumor or aneurysm of cerebral arteries. Congenital defects in the formation of ventricles can also predispose to this. Tumor of cells that produce the CSF can increase the formation of CSF and predispose to hydrocephalus.

Caution and Recommendations to Therapists:

In infants with hydrocephalus, rhythmic stroking and holding has a positive effect emotionally. The gentle, repetitive and rhythmic strokes also help reduce the spasticity of the muscles. Rhythmic movements that are slow and relaxed with the hand broad and flat are very effective. The skin over the head and face are very fragile and break down easily. Use very gentle strokes. While changing position reduce the strain on the neck by moving the head, neck and shoulders simultaneously as the body. In adults, the aim is to reduce the spasticity and prevent contractures. Passively move all joints. Gently stretch the spastic muscles. Do not use force. Start with 15 minute sessions and then proceed to a longer duration. If treating after surgery, avoid area of incision.

Notes: _____

It is treated with surgery that shunts the excess fluid from the ventricles of the brain to the atrium of the heart or into the abdominal cavity.

Hyperaldosteronism (Conn's syndrome)

Endocrine system

A condition where there is increased secretion of the steroidal hormone aldosterone from the adrenal cortex.

Cause:

It is usually caused by growth of an aldosterone secreting tumor in the adrenal cortex. In some cases the cause is unknown. Other conditions that reduce the volume of fluid or sodium in the blood vessels can also produce increased secretion of aldosterone.

Signs and Symptoms:

The symptoms are due to excess sodium and water retained in the body and decreased potassium. The expanded volume of fluid overloads the heart and can lead to hypertension and cardiac failure. Decreased potassium makes the muscles and nerves hyperirritable. There is muscle weakness, fatigue and headache. The sensations are reduced. Diabetes mellitus is common in these individuals as the low potassium level interferes with the secretion of insulin.

Risk factors:

See Cause

Caution and Recommendations to Therapists:

Massage is not contraindicated. Take a detailed history. The massage techniques have to be altered on an individual basis according to presenting symptoms.

Notes: _____

This endocrine disorder is managed by surgery or by administration of drugs that retain potassium and at the same time increase water and sodium excretion by the kidneys. Dietary salt intake is also restricted.

Aldosterone regulates the level of sodium and water along with antidiuretic hormone of the posterior pituitary gland. Aldosterone reduces the excretion of water and sodium, and increases the excretion of potassium from the body, by having a direct effect on the tubules of the kidney.

Hyperparathyroidism Endocrine system

A condition where there is overactivity of the parathyroid gland with secretion of excess parathormone.

Cause:

It is usually caused by a tumor in the parathyroid gland. Increased secretion also occurs when there is a deficiency of vitamin D or renal failure.

Signs and Symptoms:

The high levels of calcium in the blood promote stone formation in the kidneys. The rapid absorption of calcium from the bone causes thinning of bones and tendency to fracture. Bone pain, and low back pain are common symptoms. Severe abdominal pain, formation of peptic ulcers are other associated problems. The muscle atrophies and is weak. Psychological problems such as depression, personality disturbances are also seen.

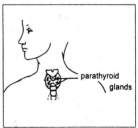
parathyroid glands

Risk factors:

See Cause.

Caution and Recommendations to Therapists:

The thinning of bones makes the client very vulnerable to fractures. Techniques using very light strokes are the only type of massage that should be employed till the underlying condition is treated. Encourage client to drink large volumes of water.

Notes: ──

Parathormone is one of the important regulators of calcium and phosphate metabolism and maintains the normal levels of calcium in the blood. Parathormone causes calcium to be absorbed into the blood from the bone and gut and reduces its excretion by the kidney. It is secreted by the 4 parathyroid glands that are located on the posterior aspect of the thyroid gland.

Calcium is one of the important elements required by the body. Some of the more important functions of calcium are for muscle contraction, transmission of impulses through nerves and for blood clotting.

Hyperpituitarism (Acromegaly, Gigantism)

Endocrine system

A condition where there is an increased production of human growth hormone by the anterior pituitary gland.

Cause:

It is caused by a tumor in the anterior pituitary. The cause of the tumor is not known.

Signs and Symptoms:

If the overproduction occurs before puberty, there is abnormal lengthening of the bones resulting in an unusual height of the person (gigantism). Overproduction after puberty when the epiphysial plates of the bone have been fused, results in thickening of bones, overgrowth of cartilage and connective tissue. Typically, there is protrusion of the jaw (acromegaly) with coarsening of the facial features - thick ears and nose. The enlarging tumor in the skull produces pressure symptoms - headache, vomiting. The proximity of the enlarging pituitary gland to the optic nerve causes deterioration of sight. Other effects of the overproduction of growth hormone includes osteoporosis, hypertension and diabetes mellitus. The high levels of cholesterol in the blood, due to the excess hormone causes atherosclerosis - thickening of the arterial wall and narrowing of lumen. Psychological disturbances may also occur.

Risk factors:

Rarely, there may be a family history of overproduction.

146

Caution and Recommendations to Therapists:

Massage is not contraindicated and may be beneficial to alleviate the stress produced by the sudden body change. Headaches due to this condition cannot be relieved by massage. Suspect increased intracranial pressure when a client with no history of headache suddenly develops one associated with vomiting. Encourage client to see a physician if typical signs and symptoms are seen. Emphasize the importance of following the physicians' orders regarding hormone replacement therapy after surgery.

Notes: —————————————————————————————————————

Treatment is surgical with removal of the tumor. After surgery, the person may require replacement of various hormones produced by the endocrine glands whose secretions are controlled by the pituitary.

Hypertension (High blood pressure)

Cardiovascular, Renal, Endocrine systems

A person is said to be hypertensive if the systolic blood pressure is 140 mmHg or higher and the diastolic pressure is 90 mm Hg or higher consistently.

Cause:

In primary or essential hypertension there is no evidence of other diseases. In secondary hypertension, kidney disorders may be associated. Secondary hypertension may also be due to acute brain lesions which raise the intracranial pressure. Alterations in endocrine function and hormone levels as in increased activity of adrenal cortex and medulla can also cause hypertension. Vascular disorders like arteriosclerosis or coarctation of the aorta are other causes of high blood pressure. A person is said to have malignant hypertension if the complications are rapidly progressive.

Signs and Symptoms:

Essential or primary hypertension is asymptomatic and diagnosis is made by chance. Early morning headache located in the back of the head or neck may be a symptom. Other complaints may be related to the complications in other systems. Complications include heart failure, atherosclerosis, aneurysms, angina, retinal changes and stroke.

Risk factors:

Hypertention is more common in African-Americans. Family history, advancing age, high salt intake, obesity, excess alcohol consumption, stress and use of oral contraceptives are other risk factors.

Hypertension is seen in 10% of all pregnancies.

Caution and Recommendations to Therapists:

Massage helps reduce blood pressure by relaxing the client and lowering stress. The sympathetic nervous system is also inhibited by massage. Sometimes, massage can reduce the blood pressure so much that the client can experience giddiness on getting off the massage table - postural hypotension. Clients on anti-hypertensives are also more prone to postural hypotension. The therapist should make sure that these clients get up slowly from the table, sit for some time before getting off. This enables the regulatory mechanisms of blood pressure to come into play effectively against gravity which tends to pool the blood towards the leg.

Get brochures from your local Hypertension Society and have it handy for your clients to read. Encourage clients to get their blood pressure and cholesterol levels checked regularly. Refer to Appendix IV for resources.

Notes: ────────────────────────────────

Hyperthyroidism (Thyrotoxicosis, Grave's disease, Basedow's disease, Parry's disease)

Endocrine system

A condition resulting from overproduction of thyroid hormones.

Cause:

Grave's disease, a form of hyperthyroidism, is caused by the production of antibodies that resemble the thyroid stimulating hormone of the pituitary. The thyroid stimulating hormone stimulates the thyroid gland to produce thyroxin. There is a tendency of members of a family to have this disease. Hyperthyroidism may also be caused by tumors of the thyroid gland.

Signs and Symptoms:

Symptoms are exaggerations of the normal function of the thyroid hormones (see

Notes), and resemble hyperactivity of the sympathetic system. Classically, the thyroid gland is enlarged (goiter) and appears as a swelling in front of the neck. Thyroxine excess makes the person irritable and nervous. In spite of increased appetite and intake of food, there is loss of weight. Hyperactivity of the gut causes diarrhea. Sweating, intolerance to heat, tremors, rapid heart rate are some of the typical symptoms. The accumulation of fluid and connective tissue behind the eye ball causes the eyes to bulge out (exophthalmus) in most people with hyperthyroidism. The blood vessels to the skin are dilated to dissipate the excess heat produced by the rapid metabolism and the skin appears red and flushed. There is atrophy, weakness and fatigue of muscles. The menstrual cycle is irregular in females.

Risk factors:

See Cause. Grave's disease is more common in women between the ages of 20 and 40.

Caution and Recommendations to Therapists:

Encourage client to take medications regularly.

Notes:

The thyroid gland secretes thyroxine (T4) and triiodothyronine (T3) which require iodine for formation. These hormones are necessary for normal growth and development. They increase the metabolic activity of most tissues.

Hyperthyroidism is treated with drugs, radioactive iodine and/or surgery.

Hypervitaminoses - Vitamin A and D

Endocrine system

Excessive accumulation of Vitamin A/D in the body.

Cause:

It usually results from excessive intake of supplement vitamins.

Signs and Symptoms:

Excess intake of vitamin A can cause irritability, loss of hair, headache, itching, loss of appetite, bone pain, fragility of bone, peeling and dryness of skin. The skin ear yellow or orange. In Vitamin D excess, the person has nausea, loss of appetite, loss of weight, headache, excessive urination and thirst.

....ors:

See Cause.

Caution and Recommendations to Therapists:

Encourage clients to take a well balanced diet, in which case vitamin supplements are unwarranted. Educate clients about the existence of such a condition as hypervitaminosis.

Notes: _____

See under Vitamin A and D for recommended dietary allowance.

Hypoadrenalism (Adrenal hypofunction, Adrenal insufficiency, Addison's disease)

Endocrine system

A condition where there is a decreased secretion of hormones from the adrenal cortex ie. decreased blood levels of corticosteroid, aldosterone and androgen.

Cause:

It is commonly due to destruction of the adrenal cortex by an autoimmune reaction. Antibodies produced by the body fail to recognize the tissue of the adrenal cortex as self and destroy it. Rarely, infections or lack of blood supply to the adrenals can cause this. Since the adrenal cortical secretion is regulated by the adrenocorticotrophic hormone (ACTH) secreted by the anterior pituitary, lack of ACTH can result in this condition.

In individuals treated with corticosteroids on a long term basis for other diseases, abrupt stoppage of the therapy can cause this. This is because of the atrophy of the adrenal glands and suppression of ACTH by the externally administered steroids.

Signs and Symptoms:

Typically, it produces weakness, fatigue, loss of weight and gastrointestinal symptoms like vomiting, diarrhea and loss of appetite. There is excessive pigmentation of the skin and the person looks tanned with darkening of the elbows, creases of the palms and foot and previous scars. This is because of the excess ACTH and melanocyte stimulating hormone (secreted by the pituitary) in order to stimulate the adrenals to start functioning adequately. The person is prone to postural hypotension and the pulse is weak and irregular.

The person is intolerant to even mild stress. There is a craving for salty food (loss of sodium and water due to lack of aldosterone). The decrease in androgen presents as changes in menstruation and lack of sex drive.

Risk factors:

See Cause.

Caution and Recommendations to Therapists:

Do not massage without clearance from a physician. Apart from a tendency to have postural hypotension, these individuals can go into an adrenal crisis where there is severe weakness, fatigue, nausea, vomiting, low blood pressure, dehydration and finally collapse. It can lead to kidney failure, coma and death. Also, the individuals are unable to withstand any form of stress.

Notes:

Hypoadrenalism is treated by lifelong hormonal replacement.

The adrenal cortex secretes steroidal hormones. The rate of secretion is regulated by ACTH from the anterior pituitary.

Hypoparathyroidism Endocrine system

A decreased secretion of parathormone from the parathyroid glands.

Cause:

Hypoparathyroidism may be caused by accidental removal or injury to the parathyroid gland during thyroid surgery or radiation therapy to thyroid. Rarely, the function may be depressed by antibodies formed by the body (autoimmunity).

Signs and Symptoms:

There are no symptoms in mild forms. The symptoms are related to the role of calcium in the body. The muscles become hyperirritable and go into spasm. There is tingling in the fingertips and feet. The skin is scaly and dry, with the fingernails brittle. The teeth tends to stain and decay easily. The rhythm of the heart becomes irregular and rapid.

Risk factors:

See Cause.

Caution and Recommendations to Therapists:

Encourage client to take calcium rich diets. Use massage oil liberally as the skin is scaly and dry.

Notes: ──

See notes under hyperparathyroidism. This condition is treated with calcium and vitamin D supplements.

Hypopituitarism (Panhypopituitarism, Dwarfism)

Endocrine system

A condition where there is decreased secretion of hormones by the pituitary with resultant hyposecretion from other endocrine glands regulated by it (panhypopituitarism).

Cause:

The most common cause is a tumor. Rarely, the blood supply to the pituitary is compromised in women who have extensive hemorrhage soon after delivery. Brain surgery, exposure to radiation are other rare causes. Lack of regulatory hormones from the hypothalamus (which controls the secretions by the pituitary) can also be responsible for this condition.

Signs and Symptoms:

This is related to the inadequate levels of various hormones secreted by the pituitary (see notes). The symptoms develop slowly resulting in dwarfism in children. In males, the external genitalia are underdeveloped with a small penis. In females, the menstrual cycles are absent. In both sexes, there is no or underdevelopment of pubic and axillary hair. If the onset is in adulthood, infertility, cessation of menstrual cycle, impotence are seen due to the hyposecretion from the ovaries and testis. The decreased thyroid secretion presents as lethargy, intolerance to cold, dry and thickened skin, and menstrual disturbances - all signs of hypothyroidism. The lowered levels of hormones from the adrenal cortex causes hypoglycemia, loss of appetite, hypotension and abdominal pain.

Other symptoms of increased intracranial pressure are produced if it is caused by a growing tumor. Sudden onset of headache associated with vomiting, loss of sight are some of the symptoms.

Risk factors:

See cause.

Caution and Recommendations to Therapists:

A detailed history should be obtained in order to identify the extent of the hormonal insufficiency. Encourage client to take the replacement hormones without fail. While massaging, ensure that the client is well covered (intolerance to cold may be present). Use oil liberally during massage as the skin is likely to be dry (hypothyroid symptoms). Make sure that the client changes position slowly and sits on the table for a while before getting off after massage (they may have postural hypotension). Range of motion exercises are very useful as arthritis is common. Due to the fluctuating levels of glucose these clients are prone for hypo or hyperglycemia. Keep glucose/sugar handy. Ensure that the address of a treating physician and a contact address is recorded in your clinic.

Notes: ──

The anterior pituitary secretes adrenocorticotrophic hormone (ACTH) - affects the adrenal cortex secretion; thyroid stimulating hormone (TSH) - affects thyroid gland secretion; follicle stimulating hormone (FSH) and luteinizing hormone (LH) - affects hormonal secretion from the ovaries and testis; growth hormone (GH) - affects overall growth; and prolactin - affects milk production in lactating women.

The posterior pituitary secretes Antidiuretic hormone (ADH) also known as Vasopressin - affects the concentration of body fluids by regulating the excretion of water by the kidney. It also causes the blood vessels to constrict thus increasing blood pressure. Oxytocin is another hormone secreted by the posterior pituitary. This stimulates the contraction of the uterus during labor and is also responsible for the expulsion of milk while breast-feeding.

Hypotension

A term given to blood pressure that is lower than normal. Orthostatic or postural hypotension is the abnormal drop in pressure when a person assumes an upright posture from a supine position. A drop of 20mmHg systolic pressure or 10mmHg diastolic pressure is considered abnormal.

Cause:

The body has baroreceptors (receptors that detect changes in the stretch of blood vessels) located between the heart and brain that reflexly increase blood flow to the brain whenever the blood pressure drops in the arteries supplying the brain.

In addition, antidiuretic hormone from the posterior pituitary helps maintain the blood volume and pressure by reducing the loss of fluid in the urine. In hypotension, the regulatory mechanisms are affected in various ways.

The commonest cause of hypotension is a reduction in the blood volume due to fluid loss or depletion. Hypotension can also be seen in conditions where the sympathetic nervous system activity is not adequate.

Signs and Symptoms:

The person feels dizzy or faints on getting up from a lying position or on changing posture.

Risk factors:

Prolonged vomiting, diarrhoea, or blood loss predisposes to hypotension. Hypertensive clients on antihypertensive drugs, those on diuretics (drugs that increase the formation of urine) and those with diabetes are also prone to hypotension. Prolonged bed rest and the aging process are risk factors as they reduce the sympathetic activity and sensitivity of the baroreceptors. Disorders of the autonomic nervous system - viz. the sympathetic and parasympathetic system also predispose to hypotension.

Caution and Recommendations to Therapists:

Since massage tends to lower the blood pressure, clients with severe orthostatic hypotension - those who give a history of fainting on getting up quickly from a lying position, should be massaged in a seated posture. In general, caution all clients to get up slowly from a lying posture, preferably, sit on the table for a while and move the legs to help venous return, before getting off the table.

Notes:

Hypothyroidism (Myxedema, Cretinism)

The deficiency of thyroid hormone secretion.

Cause:

In infants, it is caused by underdevelopment of the thyroid gland. Rarely, there may be an absence of one of the enzymes required for the synthesis of thyroxine. If the mother is on antithyroid drugs for hyperthyroidism during pregnancy, it may result in hypothyroidism in the infant. In adults, hyposecretion may be a result of inflammation, infection, production of antibodies against the hormone (autoimmunity), exposure to radiation, or thyroid surgery for other reasons. Lack of adequate iodine in the diet can also result in hypothyroidism.

Signs and Symptoms:

The symptoms resemble hypoactivity of the sympathetic nervous system ie. the metabolism is slowed down. In children it results in mental retardation if left undiagnosed and untreated within the first few months after birth. The baby is inactive and sleeps excessively. Growth is slow and dwarfism results.

In adults, the person is lethargic, overweight, with intolerance to cold. The skin is dry and scaly with the hair coarse and brittle. The face, hands and legs are puffy. The heart rate is slow. Thickening of the vocal cords produces a deepening and hoarseness of voice in women. One of the complications of hypothyroidism is coma. This may be precipitated by stress.

Risk factors:

It is more common in women.

Caution and Recommendations to Therapists:

Ensure that the client is properly covered as they are intolerant to cold. Use oil liberally as the skin is coarse and dry. They are prone to osteoporosis, so excessive pressure should not be used. Abdominal massage helps relieve constipation that these individuals are prone to. Massage helps alleviate the depression, a psychological effect of the disease. Encourage client to take medications regularly. Medications are required to be taken throughout life.

Notes:

See Notes under Hyperthyroidism. Hypothyroidism is treated with hormone replacement.

Impetigo

A bacterial infection of the epidermis of the skin.

Cause:

It is caused by staphylococci or a type of streptococci (group A beta-hemolytic) bacteria.

Signs and Symptoms:

The infection may start in an apparently normal skin or superinfect a scratch or insect bite. The infection starts as a rounded, raised, fluid filled cavity in a reddened area. Soon a pustule is seen. The pustule discharges a honey colored or yellowish fluid which dries and forms a crust. New lesions appear rapidly in surrounding areas (see Appendix 1 figure: 6).

If impetigo is left untreated, complications affecting the kidney - glomerulonephritis can occur. It may also spread to the dermis to form ecthyma.

Risk factors:

It is more common in children, but adults can be infected too. It is often seen secondary to scabies.

Caution and Recommendations to Therapists:

The infection can spread by contact - especially in individuals with lowered immunity. Massage is contraindicated locally if the lesion is confined to a very small area. Make sure that the infected area is covered with a bandage and does not come in contact with you or the linen. If the lesions are extensive do not massage. Since the infection can be treated and responds well to antibiotics advise client to seek medical help. Impetigo has to be distinguished from eczema (not contagious) which typically appears as multiple patches in skin flexures.

Notes: _____

Infectious Mononucleosis (Kissing disease)

An acute viral infection primarily affecting the upper respiratory tract

Cause:

It is caused by the Epstein-Barr virus. The virus is spread through salivary secretions. It may also spread by blood transfusion. It is highly contagious and individuals are contagious even before the symptoms develop and continue to be infectious through the symptomatic phase, as well as for an indefinite period after the symptoms subside. The incubation period ranges from 10-50 days.

Signs and Symptoms:

Typically it presents with fever (higher in the evening), sore throat and enlargement of cervical lymph nodes. As the name suggests there is an increase in monocytes and lymphocytes in the blood. There may be enlargement of the spleen and liver. It may be accompanied by a rash. Jaundice may also be present. Although complications are rare, it includes splenic rupture, meningitis, encephalitis, anemia and thrombocytopenia (platelet deficiency). The symptoms subside in 6-10 days. However, in some individuals it may persist for weeks.

Risk factors:

It is more common in young adults and children. There is a higher incidence of infectious mononucleosis in the United States, Canada and Europe.

Caution and Recommendations to Therapists:

Since it is difficult to prevent and treat the disease due to its' long incubation period and persistence even after symptoms subside, avoid massaging individuals who have been diagnosed with infectious nucleosis at least until the symptoms subside (which may be a few weeks to months). Be careful while massaging the abdomen in individuals who have just recovered from the disorder as the splenic enlargement may persist. Excessive pressure may result in splenic rupture. Gentle massage with the use of heating pads help relieve persisting body ache.

Notes:

It is treated with aspirin and other forms of supportive treatment as it resists prevention and antimicrobial treatment.

Inflammatory Bowel Disease - Crohn's Disease, (IBD, Regional enteritis, Granulomatous colitis)

An inflammatory disease of the gastrointestinal tract affecting all layers of the intestinal wall.

Cause:

The exact cause is not known. Immune disorders and allergies have been implicated. The blockage of lymphatic flow in the gut leads to edema, inflammation, ulceration, healing by fibrosis, infection and abscess formation. The wall eventually thickens and has the appearance of a hose. The commonest region to be affected is the ileum (last part of the small intestine). However, any region from the mouth to the anus can be affected.

Signs and Symptoms:

Initially, the symptoms are vague with mild pain in the abdomen. The symptoms vary according to the location affected and can range from fever and nausea to flatulence and diarrhoea. There may be blood in the stools. In chronic cases, the person has diarrhea, pain in the lower right quadrant of the abdomen, loss of weight, and fatty, foul smelling stools. Other signs of malabsorption are also there (see malabsorption syndrome). The symptoms may be altered by complications of stricture formation. Fistulas (abnormal communications between two structures) between the intestine and other areas like bladder or the surface of the skin may form. Formation of abscess is also common. The disease progresses with remissions and exacerbations.

Risk factors:

It is more common between the ages of 20-40. There is a genetic predisposition with higher incidence in those with a family history. It is also common in Jews. Stress can make the symptoms worse. Crohn's affects men and women equally.

Caution and Recommendations to Therapists:

The aim of the massage is to reduce stress and relax the client.

Avoid massage over the abdominal area during a flare-up of the condition. In general, deep or vigorous treatment of the abdomen and back should be avoided.

Since these clients may be on corticosteroids and drugs that suppress immunity, they are prone to infection. Do not treat if you have even a mild infection.

The malnutrition due to malabsorption, makes their skin bruise easily. Do not use excessive pressure. The skin is dry due to poor nutrition as well as dehydration. The oil used for massage may be helpful.

Clients with this condition are also prone to osteoporosis, reiterating that only light pressure should be used. Encourage them to keep a close watch on the kind of diet that triggers or worsens symptoms. Frequent small meals are helpful. Advice client to increase the intake of water to two to three liters per day. Encourage clients to join local support groups. See Appendix IV for resources.

Notes: _____

The treatment for this condition is symptomatic. The malabsorption is compensated with intravenous supplements. Steroids and drugs that suppress immunity are also given along with anti-inflammatory drugs. Surgery is done to reduce symptoms in severe cases. Here, portions of the affected gut is cut and joined with normal bowel. In severe cases, the ileum is opened on to the surface of the abdominal wall (ileostomy).

Inflammatory Bowel Diseases may be associated with arthritis and muscle pain.

Inflammatory Bowel Disease (IBD)

- Ulcerative colitis   Gastrointestinal system

A chronic inflammatory disease of the gastrointestinal tract primarily affecting the superficial (mucosal) layer of the large intestines.

Cause:

The cause is not known. It is said to be caused by an abnormal immune response in the gastrointestinal tract. The inflammation of the mucosa of the colon and rectum results in ulceration of the mucosa and thickening of the gut.

Signs and Symptoms:

The symptoms are seen as remissions and exacerbations and can be of varying severity. Diarrhoea, blood and mucus in stools, abdominal pain, fever are some of the symptoms seen. Signs of malabsorption and malnutrition like weight loss and fatigue are often seen. The person may have arthritis.

Risk factors:

Women are more commonly affected. It is commoner between the second and third decade of life with a higher incidence in Caucasians.

Caution & Recommendations to Therapist:

Similar to Crohn's disease (see Inflammatory Bowel Disease - Crohn's disease).

Notes: ────────────────────────────────

(see Inflammatory Bowel Disease - Crohn's disease) There is a higher incidence of cancer in people with ulcerative colitis.

═══

Influenza (Grippe, Flu)

Respiratory system

A highly contagious respiratory tract infection.

Cause:

It is a viral infection produced by different strains of three different types of Myxovirus influenzae. It is transmitted by inhalation of the droplets expelled into the air as infected individuals cough or sneeze. It may also spread by sharing glasses with an infected person. The virus enters the system through the respiratory epithelium and produces an inflammatory response.

Signs and Symptoms:

It takes 1-2 days after infection for symptoms to be produced. There is a sudden onset of fever with chills, headache, dry cough, body ache, laryngitis, congestion and watery discharge from nose and eyes. There may be enlargement of the cervical lymph node enlargement. Fatigue and general weakness may persist for weeks even though the acute symptoms subside in a few days. Complications like pneumonia, worsening of obstructive pulmonary disease (if present) may occur. Rarely, it may lead to pericarditis and nervous system complications like encephalitis.

Risk factors:

It is more common in the colder months. The symptoms are more severe in young children, the elderly, immunocompromised individuals and those with other chronic diseases.

Caution and Recommendations to Therapists:

Be informed about outbreaks of influenza in your area. It may be wise to have annual inoculations of flu vaccines (not advisable if pregnant) at the start of the flu season ie. in late autumn. Do not massage clients with influenza until they have fully recovered. Therapists with influenza should not massage clients until all symptoms have disappeared. Proper disposal of tissues, hand washing, covering mouth while sneezing or coughing are simple techniques that can prevent spread of disease.

Notes: _____

Influenza vaccine is reformulated every year according to the type of virus that is likely to affect the society. Side effects of vaccination is usually restricted to local irritation and fever for a short duration.

Intestinal obstruction — Gastrointestinal system

The impairment of movement of the contents of the intestine in the direction of the rectum and anus.

Cause:

The obstruction could be due to mechanical reasons or due to paralysis of the autonomic system. Mechanically, the lumen of the intestine can be obstructed by hernias, growths, strictures (common in ulcerative colitis), foreign bodies like gall stones, worms, fruit pits and adhesions between organs (can occur after abdominal surgery). Rarely, the gut can telescope onto itself (intussusception) or twist on itself (volvulus) causing obstruction.

Paralysis and loss of all movements of the bowel usually occurs after abdominal surgery (paralytic ileus). However, paralytic ileus is temporary and disappears after 2-3 days. It can also occur after back injuries and spinal cord injuries or thrombosis in the vessels that supply the gut.

Signs and Symptoms:

There is abdominal distention due to the accumulation of fluids and gases. Constipation, colicky abdominal pain and vomiting are also present. The obstruction perpetuates the growth of bacteria. The toxins produced by bacteria and death of tissue, is absorbed into the blood resulting in further complications. The loss of fluid leads to symptoms of dehydration - reduced urine formation, dry and loose skin texture and intense thirst. There is weakness, excessive sweating and anxiety.

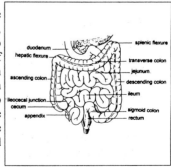

Risk factors:

It can be a complication of hernia or abdominal surgery.

Caution and Recommendations to Therapists:

Do not massage if intestinal obstruction is suspected. Refer to a physician immediately.

Notes:

Intussuseption, volvulus, strangulation of herniated gut and other acute obstructions require emergency surgery as they can be fatal.

Jaundice (Icterus)　　　Gastrointestinal, Cardiovascular system

(French: jaune - yellow)

The yellow discoloration of the skin due to abnormally high levels of the pigment bilirubin in the blood.

Cause:

Bilirubin is a breakdown product of hemoglobin of the red blood cells. It is metabolized in the liver and secreted in the bile along with the bile salts. Therefore, any condition that increases the breakdown of red blood cells, or affects its metabolism in the liver, or retards its excretion in the bile can result in abnormal increase of bilirubin in the blood. Thus jaundice can be classified as prehepatic, hepatic or posthepatic according to the cause.

Signs and Symptoms:

Bilirubin has an affinity for elastic tissue and usually presents as a yellow discoloration of the white of the eye. Mucous membranes of the mouth also appear yellow. In prehepatic jaundice, there will be associated anemia. History of hepatitis along with other signs of hepatitis will be present in the hepatic type (see Hepatitis). There may be severe itching of the skin especially in the posthepatic type of jaundice. In addition, in the latter, due to the obstruction to the flow of bile, digestion of fat is affected and the feces is foul smelling and clay colored due to the lack of bile. The urine is dark in color as a result of increased excretion of bilirubin in the urine.

Risk factors:

Transfusion of incompatible blood, hereditary disorders of the red blood cells like sickle cell anemia, thalassemia and spherocytosis predispose to prehepatic jaundice.

Hepatic jaundice is the most common type and is due to viral hepatitis. This type can also be caused by liver failure due to toxic agents, drugs, cirrhosis or cancer. Rarely, hereditary absence of liver enzymes required for the metabolism of bilirubin can predispose an individual to jaundice.

Bile duct abnormalities, gall stones or tumors obstructing the flow of bile can predispose an individual to posthepatic jaundice.

Caution and Recommendations to Therapists:

The cause of the jaundice should dictate the treatment plan. Prehepatic jaundice is not contagious and can be treated on an individual basis. A soothing massage of short duration is indicated. Avoid massage to the upper abdomen as both the spleen and the liver are likely to be enlarged in these individuals. The massage should be gentle and soothing. Undue pressure should not be used as the individual may have a bleeding disorder and bruises and bleeds easily.

The cause of hepatic jaundice should be obtained. If due to Viral Hepatitis, the precautions given under hepatitis should be followed.

If the jaundice is posthepatic, the massage oil may reduce the intense itching experienced by these individuals. Massage to the abdomen should be avoided.

Notes: ──

Those with prehepatic jaundice may require frequent blood transfusions. Supportive treatment is given for hepatic jaundice. Posthepatic jaundice is usually treated surgically.

The metabolism of bilirubin.

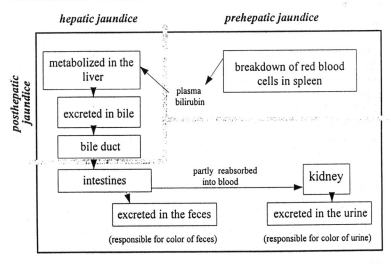

Kyphosis

A deformity of the spine that produces a rounded back.

Cause:

In children and adolescents it is due to bad posture. It may be also be brought about by arthritis, lung problems like emphysema, paralysis or weakness of back muscles.

Signs and Symptoms:

The back is rounded and the chest flattened. There may be difficulty in breathing due to the shortening of the pectoral muscles that interferes with thoracic movement. The rhomboids, trapezius and the longitudinal muscles of the back are stretched and weakened. The scapula is pulled forward and the person has a forward head posture.

Risk factors:

Occupations that require a hunched posture can predispose to kyphosis.

Caution and Recommendations to Therapists:

Work in close conjunction with the physiotherapist and physician.

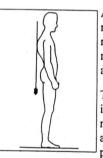

A proper assessment is required to identify the extent of spasm, range of motion, trigger points and adhesions. The trapezius, rhomboids, latissimus dorsi, erector spinae, pectoralis minor and major are some of the muscles that have to be tested for strength and length.

The aim is to produce general relaxation, reduce pain by increasing circulation in the tense muscles, and stretch shortened muscles and fascia. Position the client in as comfortable posture as possible with supporting pillows. Heat packs may help reduce pain and spasm. Start with the client supine and use techniques to stretch the shortened pectorals. Massage the tense neck and pectoral muscles addressing trigger points if present. In the prone position, use techniques to stimulate the rhomboids and trapezius. The rotator cuff muscles, gluteal and back muscles should also be massaged thoroughly.

Deep diaphragmatic breathing helps mobilize the thoracic cavity. The client should be encouraged to do remedial exercises to mobilize the joints and strengthen weak muscles. Avoid mobilizing techniques if the kyphosis is due to changes in bone or connective tissue.

Notes: _____

Kyphosis is classified as *primary, functional* or *first degree* if the deformity is of muscular origin and can be corrected; *secondary, structural* or *second degree* if due to connective tissue change and *tertiary* or *third degree* if due to bony changes.

Laryngitis

An inflammation of the vocal cords.

Cause:

It is usually caused by viral or bacterial infection. Excessive use of the voice can also produce this condition.

Signs and Symptoms:

It presents with hoarseness or complete loss of voice, cough and pain on swallowing.

Risk factors:

It is more common in occupations like teaching, public speaking or singing. Loud cheering, constant dust, smoke or fume inhalation, smoking and alcoholism are other predisposing conditions.

Caution and Recommendations to Therapists:

If the laryngitis is due to viral or bacterial infection it spreads by inhalation of droplets from the infected person. Do not massage clients with laryngitis of infective origin. Encourage rest to the voice. Increase humidification of air, reduce air conditioning (which tends to dehumidify) while treating clients with laryngitis of noninfective origin.

Notes:

Leukemia

A cancerous multiplication of white blood cells in the bone marrow and lymph tissue with abnormally large number of white blood cells in the blood.

Cause:

It may be due to certain viruses. But family history, exposure to radiation and certain chemicals have also been associated with this disease. The immature white blood cells seem to multiply abnormally in the area of origin: lymphatic tissue - lymphocytes, bone marrow - other white blood cells. They then spill over into the blood and other organs affecting their normal function.

Signs and Symptoms:

It may present as a sudden onset of fever and abnormal bleeding from the nose, gums or other regions. The individual is also more prone to bruise easily. There may be mild fever, weight loss, and fatigue lasting for a number of days. Even though the number of white blood cells are increased they are immature with lowered function, so there is a tendency to have repeated infections. The rapid multiplication in the bones may also produce bone pain.

Risk factors:

Family history, Down's syndrome, exposure to radiation, occupation involving exposure to benzene are all predisposing factors.

Caution and Recommendations to Therapists:

Do not massage a client diagnosed with leukemia without consulting the treating physician. However, since the problem is in the circulating blood and tissues producing blood cells, there is little chance of spreading the condition to other areas by massaging. These clients are more prone to infection due to the lowered immunity. Even if the physician approves a massage, do not treat clients if you have even a mild infection. Ensure that they are scheduled for a time when they are unlikely to come in contact with infected individuals. These clients also bruise easily and have a tendency to bleed. Do not use excess pressure. Use ice packs in areas that have bled or bleed. There may be enlargement of spleen or liver. Avoid massaging the upper abdominal region ie. over the liver and spleen. Only a very gentle relaxation massage should be given. Avoid areas of radiation if the person is on radiation therapy. Refer client to local support groups (see Appendix IV).

Notes:

Leukemias are classified according to the speed of onset as acute or chronic leukemias. The type with increase in lymphocytes are called lympho-blastic/lymphocytic leukemias. The type with increase in other white blood cells are called myeloblastic leukemias. Those producing increase in monocytes are called monocytic/monoblastic leukemias. Thus there could be an acute or chronic type of each of the above. The age group they affect and the progress of each of the types vary. Leukemias are generally treated with chemotherapy and/or radiation.

Lichen Planus

(Greek: tree moss)

An inflammatory skin disorder.

Cause:

The cause is unknown.

Signs and Symptoms:

It presents as itchy, small, papular lesions which appear like tree moss in the wrist, ankles and trunk. The eruptions glisten and appear as white lines or spots.

Risk factors:

It may be associated with drugs and chemicals like arsenic, bismuth and gold.

Caution and Recommendations to Therapists:

It is not contagious. Chemicals in the oil used may make the condition worse so unadulterated oil should be used while massaging such clients.

Notes:

The lesions may disappear spontaneously. It is treated symptomatically and drugs are given to relieve the itching. Sometimes steroids are used.

Liver Failure

A condition when the liver is unable to cope up with the demands made.

Cause:

Any condition that extensively damages the hepatic tissue leads to liver failure. Only 10% of the liver is required for the liver to function.

Signs and Symptoms:

These are related to the various functions that the liver performs. Due to the lack of clotting factors, the person bleeds easily and anemia results. The congestion of the portal circulation can lead to fluid in the peritoneal cavity (ascites), edema and varicosities of esophageal and rectal vessels - potential sites of fatal bleeding (see esophageal varices).

The inadequate metabolism of steroid hormones is reflected as menstrual irregularities, impotence and sterility. There is atrophy of the testis and abnormal enlargement of the breasts in men. Jaundice is also present. The increase in toxins in the blood can affect the nervous system causing lack of mental alertness, confusion, coma and convulsions.

Risk factors:

Hepatitis, cirrhosis and ingestion of drugs toxic to the liver, alcoholism and prolonged obstruction to the bile ducts can predispose to liver failure.

Caution and Recommendations to Therapists:

The cause of the liver failure should be determined before proceeding. Treatment is altered according to the cause. See hepatitis, cirrhosis and portal hypertension for specific recommendations.

Notes: ————————————————————————

Liver transplant is one of the newer treatment options. Those who have had transplants are required to be on immunosuppressants to prevent the body from rejecting the donor tissue. Hence these individuals are prone to infections.

Lung Abscess

A lung infection associated with accumulation of pus.

Cause:

It may be caused by different types of bacteria. Rarely, it may be caused by an amoeba or a fungus. Lung abscess may occur as a complication of bronchopneumonia and other lung infections. It is also associated with aspiration of contents of the mouth and pharynx.

Signs and Symptoms:

Cough with foul-smelling or blood-tinged sputum, chest pain produced by breathing movements, difficulty in breathing, fever and weight loss are the classical symptoms.

Risk factors:

The incidence is higher in people with poor oral hygiene ie. those with dental or gum diseases. Coma, general anaesthesia, repeated vomiting, bronchial obstruction by tumors or thick secretions, chronic upper respiratory tract infections, individuals with difficulty in swallowing as a result of muscle weakness or cranial nerve damage are prone.

Caution and Recommendations to Therapists:

Individuals with lung abscess have to be on antibiotic treatment often lasting for months. Consult physician before treating. Postural drainage is beneficial (see bronchiectasis). Tapotement, chest hacking and vibration movements help with drainage of pus. Deep breathing exercises also help. Steam inhalation before commencing treatment in a person recovering from lung abscess may be beneficial.

Notes: _____

Lyme Disease (Lyme arthritis)

Nervous, Cardiovascular, Musculoskeletal, Integumentary systems

An inflammatory infectious disease transmitted by ticks, that affects many systems.

Cause:

This disease is caused by a bacteria that is carried by ticks. The life cycle of the tick spans over two years and has three stages - larvae, nymph and adult. In North America, the mouse carries the larvae and nymph and the white-tailed deer the adult tick. All stages can feed on humans. It is necessary for the infected tick to be attached to the human body for 24 hours for the infection to be transmitted.

Signs and Symptoms:

Within an few days or a month after the tick bite, the bacteria moves to the surface of the skin producing a circular, ring-like rash that has red borders with central clearing. The person also has flu-like symptoms - fever, headache, fatigue and enlargement of lymph nodes. If it is not treated, the bacteria migrates to the other systems through the lymph or blood. Complications like meningitis and arthritis may result.

Risk factors:

It is common in North America, Europe and Asia.

Caution and Recommendations to Therapists:

This disease spreads only by tick bites and there is no danger of spread through massage. Since the disease is chronic - lasting for months to years, the massage treatment has to be individualized according to symptoms. Encourage client to see physician and take the full course of antibiotics prescribed.

Notes:

This disease can be prevented by avoiding tick infested areas from May to October. Exposure of the skin should be reduced by suitable clothings while moving through heavily wooded areas.

Application of insect repellent and removal of ticks within a few hours of attachment prevents the disease.

Lymphangitis Lymphatic system

Inflammation of lymphatic vessels.

Cause:

It is usually caused by the streptococci bacteria.

Signs and Symptoms:

There is pain and swelling of the affected area accompanied by enlargement of lymph nodes, inflammation of the lymph vessels and fever. The inflamed vessels appear as red streaks on the skin.

Risk factors:

It usually spreads from infection in other areas.

Caution and Recommendations to Therapists:

The therapist can get infected by contact, if open wounds are present.

Massage is contraindicated. Massage can exacerbate the illness and also help spread the infection to other areas or to the rest of the body (septicemia). Advice clients to see a physician if not seeing one already. Encourage client to take the full course of antibiotics.

Notes:

Malabsorption syndrome Gastrointestinal system

The spectrum of symptoms and signs seen when there is failure to absorb nutrients from the intestinal tract.

Cause:

This can be caused by reduced or no secretion of enzymes required for digestion and absorption of a specific type of food, or defect in the mucosa which transports the digested food from the lumen of the intestine to the blood for distribution, or due to lymphatic obstruction in the gut. Reduced secretion occurs if the glands like the pancreas, liver etc. are dysfunctional. It can also occur if the normal growth of the bacteria in the gut have been disturbed.

No absorption occurs through the mucosa if there are lesions in it as in Crohn's disease or if a large portion of the gut has been removed by surgery. This may also occur if the intestinal villi are atrophied as in a condition called Celiac sprue (Celiac Disease). Sprue is due to an immunological reaction to a certain protein called gluten contained in barley, wheat and rye.

Since the lymphatics transport fat in the gut, fat absorption is disturbed if the lymphatics are obstructed as in trauma, infections or cancer.

Signs and Symptoms:

These individuals present with diarrhea, fatty, foul smelling stools that float in the toilet and are difficult to flush, abdominal pain, bloated abdomen and flatulence (passage of gas). There is weight loss in spite of a normal intake of food. Other signs seen are due to the lack of absorption of vitamins (see vitamin deficiencies).

Risk factors:

Celiac sprue has a genetic predisposition and affects Caucasians.

Caution and Recommendations to Therapists:

Due to the lack of vitamins, the skin is dry and scaly. The oil used for massage is therefore beneficial. Due to the lack of vitamin K, the individuals bruise very easily and moderate pressure can cause bleeding under the skin. So very light pressure should be used. The lack of vitamin D makes them prone to osteoporosis - reiterating the use of only mild pressure during massage. Lack of vitamin B can produce alteration in sensations especially in the distal parts of the limbs - so the client may not be able to give adequate feedback. Protein deficiency can produce edema. Lymphatic drainage techniques may be used if edema is present. Gentle abdominal massage can help relieve the gas that produces the distension and discomfort. Refer client to local support groups (see Appendix IV for resources).

Notes: _____

Malabsorption syndrome is treated with supplements that are given intravenously.

Malignant Lymphomas (Non-Hodgkin's Lymphoma, Lymphosarcoma)

Lymphatic system

A cancer originating in the lymph nodes and other lymphoid tissues.

Cause:

The cause is unknown. It may be due to a virus.

Signs and Symptoms:

Initially, it presents as swelling of the lymph nodes, tonsils, adenoids, liver or spleen. The swelling is painless and the nodes feel rubbery. As the swelling increases in size it produces symptoms by pressure on surrounding areas accompanied by anemia, weight loss, fever, lethargy and fatigue.

Risk factors:

It is more common in males and occurs in all age groups. There is a higher incidence in Caucasians and Jews.

Caution and Recommendations to Therapists:

Advice the client to consult a physician if you notice an abnormally large painless lymph node enlargement. Do not massage clients diagnosed with lymphoma without consulting the treating physician.

Notes :

Lymphoma is treated with radiation and/or chemotherapy.

Marfan's Syndrome

Musculoskeletal, Cardiovascular systems

An inherited disorder producing abnormal development of elastin and collagen of the connective tissue.

Cause:

It is inherited from either of the parents and the child exhibits symptoms of the disease to varying degrees even if one parent is normal ie. it is a dominant trait. In

15% of the cases, it may be due to a fresh mutation ie. there is no family history.

Signs and Symptoms:

Most commonly, these individuals are very tall with an arm span that is longer than the height of the person. The ligaments, tendons and joint capsules are weak resulting in hyperextensibility of joints. The joints tend to get dislocated easily. Marfan's syndrome also affects the eye causing detachment of the lens and increased pressure of the ocular fluid. Bone deformities are also seen with development of pigeon chest. If the cardiovascular system is affected, the weak walls of the aorta dilate and bulge resulting in aneurysm formation with potential for rupture.

Risk factors:

See Cause.

Caution and Recommendations to Therapists:

Gentle massage is recommended. Do not use pressure or manipulative and mobilization techniques. Encourage client to take genetic counselling. Refer to local support groups, if available. See Appendix IV for resources.

Notes: ───

Measles (Rubeola)   Integumentary, Respiratory systems

A virus infection that produces rashes in the skin.

Cause:

It is caused by the measles virus. The virus is spread by air borne and droplet contact. The incubation period ranges from 1-3 weeks. The virus enters the respiratory tract and then gains access to the blood via the lymphatic system.

Signs and Symptoms:

It presents as fever, cough, watering of the eyes and congestion of the nose, 2-3 days before the development of the rash. The rash appears over the face and head as small reddish spots. Within a day the rash spreads to the arms, trunk and back. Soon, the rashes join together and present as large reddish areas. Rarely, encephalitis may occur.

174

Risk factors:

Contact with an infected individual increases the risk.

Caution and Recommendations to Therapists:

Although measles is one of the milder forms of diseases, it can have serious consequences in an individual whose immunity is low. Infected individuals should refrain from work for 5-21 days after exposure, or at least 7 days after the rash appears to ensure that they do not spread the disease.

Notes: —————————————————————————————

Measles vaccines are available. The newer vaccines have minimal side effects and are very effective in preventing the disease.

Medial tibial stress syndrome
(Tibial periostitis)   Musculoskeletal system

The inflammation of the periosteum in the distal posteromedial aspect of the tibia.

Cause:

It is caused by excessive use of the posterior tibialis and soleus muscle.

Signs and Symptoms:

This condition is similar to shin splints, but the pain is localized to the distal third of the tibia in the posteromedial aspect. The pain is felt over a discrete area about 3-6 cms in this region. The pain is increased on plantar flexing and turning the foot inwards.

Risk factors:

Exercises involving plantar flexion and inversion of foot can predispose to this condition.

Caution and Recommendations to Therapists:

In acute cases, the limb is rested for 2-3 days. Apply icepacks, and elevate limb to reduce swelling and inflammation. Later use friction massage, to increase blood flow and prevent adhesions. Gentle stretching also helps. Refer to physiotherapist for strengthening exercises.

Notes: ──

Meningitis

An inflammation of the meninges (the covering of the brain and spinal cord - pia, arachnoid and dura mater).

Cause:

It is usually caused by a bacterial infection but can be due to virus or tuberculosis. The infections often spreads from foci in other regions of the body and may follow pneumonia, osteomyelitis, ear infection, sinusitis etc. Infection may also follow fracture of the skull or invasive procedures such as lumbar puncture or neurosurgery.

Signs and Symptoms:

The person has fever with chills - the generalized symptoms of infection. Due to the inflammation in the intracranial cavity, the pressure of the cerebrospinal fluid is increased producing headache and vomiting. The person resists any movement that tends to stretch the meninges. Hence there is resistance on passively raising the leg of a person with meningitis (Kernig's sign). If the neck is flexed passively that too is resisted (Brudzinski's sign). Other symptoms include irritability, double vision, drowsiness, convulsions, confusion, delirium and coma.

Risk factors:

Prolonged untreated or inadequately treated infection in other areas of the body may predispose to meningitis. Bacterial meningitis is more common in children and the elderly.

Caution and Recommendations to Therapists:

Suspect meningitis as the cause of headache if there is a history of sudden onset of headache associated with fever and neck stiffness in a person who has never experienced such a headache before. Do not massage, but refer to a physician.

Viral meningitis can occur as a seasonal epidemic. The virus spreads through the secretions of infected individuals. Scrupulous hand washing prevents spread of disease. Be fully informed of epidemics in your area.

Notes: ───

Menigitis is treated with antibiotics, if bacterial. Other forms of treatment are supportive and include pain killers, bed rest and monitoring of fluid and electrolyte balance. The complications of meningitis may be cranial nerve damage, blockage of flow of the cerebrospinal fluid leading to hydrocephalus.

Molluscum Contagiosum (Acne varioliformis)

Integumentary system

A viral disease of the skin.

Cause:

This is a mildly contagious disease of the skin caused by a virus. It can be transmitted by skin-to-skin contact, or fomites or by self inoculation. The incubation period ranges from 1 week to 6 months.

Signs and Symptoms:

Crops of semi-globular, pin-head sized, waxy, pinkish yellow painless growths are seen on the surface of the skin. Typically, each papule has a central depression through which a cheesy secretion can be expressed. The papule slowly grows in size and may persist for months or years. Secondary infection may occur (see Appendix I figure 8). Often, treatment is not sought by clients as the condition is painless.

Risk factors:

It tends to be more common in those who are immunocompromised.

Caution and Recommendations to Therapists:

It can spread by direct contact. Avoid the area, or cover the lesions with a bandage before massaging. Since the treatment is a simple procedure, advice the client to seek a physician's help.

Notes: ────────────────────────────────────

It is treated by freezing, surgical removal of papules or by removing the top of the papule and applying sclerosing agents. It can be permanently treated.

Multiple myeloma (Malignant plasmacytoma, Plasma cell myeloma, Myelomatosis)

Musculoskeletal system

An abnormal and uncontrolled multiplication of plasma cells.

Cause:

The cause is unknown. There is abnormal multiplication of the plasma cells in the bone marrow. The tumor cells infiltrate the skeleton making them prone to pathological fractures. Later other organs of the body are infiltrated.

Signs and Symptoms:

It usually begins as a severe low back pain. Bone pain, and joint swelling may be present. Other signs are found when the weakened vertebra collapses. In late stages, symptoms related to other systems such as the renal, respiratory system are seen.

Risk factors:

It is more common in men above the age of 40.

Caution and Recommendations to Therapists:

The disease is often diagnosed after it is wide spread. Consult Physician before massage. These clients are prone to fractures due to the demineralization of bones. Only very light, superficial massage, range of motion and breathing exercises should be considered. If the client is bedridden look for pressure ulcers and avoid area.

Notes: ────────────────────────────────────

It is treated with chemotherapy and pain killers.

Multiple Sclerosis (MS)

A disorder that progressively affects the myelin sheath of the neurons in the brain and spinal cord.

Cause:

The cause is unknown. It may be due to a slow acting viral infection or due to an autoimmune response. Due to the higher prevalence in certain geographical areas, an environmental factor has been implicated. The presence of lymphocytes in the affected neurons suggest an abnormal immunological response. The white matter of the brain - where the myelin is present, is the area affected.

Signs and Symptoms:

The symptoms vary according to the area and extent of the brain and spinal cord affected. There is exacerbation and remission of the disease with the person symptom-free between the spells in the early stages of the disease. The symptoms last from hours to weeks. It initially presents as numbness and tingling sensations in different regions. Double vision and blurred vision are some of the other symptoms. Weakness, muscle paralysis affecting one or more limbs, tremors, gait problems, increased tone of muscles and exaggerated reflexes are other symptoms. Mood swings, irritability, depression may be present. In some, there may be difficulty in speech and swallowing.

Risk factors:

Studies have shown that if a person moves from an area of greater risk to a lower risk area before the age of 15, the incidence is as in the lower risk area. However, if the migration was after the age of 15, the high risk still prevails. There is also a genetic link as people in the same family are at higher risk. It is more common between the ages of 20-40 and affects more women than men. It affects Caucasians more frequently and the incidence is higher in the socioeconomic, urban population. Cold damp climate increase the risk of MS. Stress, emotional upset, extremes of temperature, can precipitate an attack.

Caution and Recommendations to Therapists:

Take time to assess the client thoroughly during *every* visit as the symptoms vary and progress unpredictability. The symptoms may change from day to day. The aim is to shorten exacerbations, relax the individual, decrease the tone in muscles which are rigid, prevent joint stiffness and contractures. Since hot or cold temperatures can make the symptoms worse, avoid using high heat or cold therapy. Mild heat helps improve circulation and decrease spasticity. Perform range of motion exercises of all joints. Use relaxing strokes while massaging rigid muscles. The strokes should be repetitive and rhythmic. Abdominal massage helps relieve constipation which is a common problem.

These clients tire easily so the duration of each session should be short in general and should be adjusted according to individual clients. Two half hour sessions per week are recommended but the treatment needs to be ongoing. Moderate exercise programs have been found to be beneficial. Since any kind of infection can precipitate an attack, and since these clients may be on corticosteroids which depresses immunity, avoid treating clients with MS when you have any kind of infection. Encourage clients to join a local support group. See Appendix IV for resources.

Notes: ────────────────────────────────

Yoga, tai chi, are other alternatives that have been found to be beneficial. Medical treatment is supportive with use of corticosteroids, plasma exchange (where the antibodies are removed) and drugs to reduce pain, spasticity and depression.

The progress of the disease is variable. In most cases, there is a relapsing and remitting course with complete or partial recovery between relapses. In some cases the course is progressive and chronic with slow continual degradation. In some, the course is acute and traumatic with severe disability within a few years.

Muscular Dystrophy (Duchenne's, Becker's, Landouzy Dejerine, Limb girdle dystrophy)

Musculoskeletal system

A group of congenital disorders that produce symmetrical wasting of skeletal muscles. There is no loss of sensation or neural activity.

Cause:

It is a genetic disorder where there is a decrease/lack of a muscle protein called dystrophin. Duchenne's and Becker's type are due to defects in the X chromosome.

Signs and Symptoms:

The degree of severity and onset of disease vary according to the type. Duchenne's begins between 3 and 5 years of age and the child may be confined to a wheelchair by age 10. The weakness of muscle starts in the leg and pelvic region. This affects the gait and posture. The muscles may give a false appearance of strength due to the bulk. The bulk is produced by replacement of muscle tissue by fibrous tissue and fat. Becker's type presents as Duchenne's, but progresses more slowly. The Facio-scapulo-humeral or Landouzy-Dejerine dystrophy weakens the muscles of the face, shoulders and upper arms initially, and then progressing to all muscles. The lips are weak and the client has difficulty whistling or puckering the mouth. The client may also have a masklike appearance. The limb-girdle type starts early (age 6) but progresses slowly, first affecting the upper arm and pelvis. The weakness may spread to the involuntary muscles and produce cardiac failure, constipation etc.

Risk factors:

Duchenne's and Becker's affect males; the other two types affect both males and females equally.

Caution and Recommendations to Therapists:

There is no cure for the disease. Move all joints actively and passively. Massage helps slow down muscle atrophy. Abdominal massage may help with the constipation that these clients suffer due to the effect of the disorder on the involuntary muscles. Clients with this disorder take a longer time to accomplish every day tasks. Be patient while the client climbs on and off table.

Keep telephone number and address of local Muscular Dystrophy Associations to refer client for emotional support and genetic counseling (see Appendix IV for resources).

Notes: ⎯⎯⎯⎯⎯⎯⎯⎯⎯⎯⎯⎯⎯⎯⎯⎯⎯⎯⎯⎯⎯⎯⎯⎯⎯⎯⎯⎯

Myositis ossificans Musculoskeletal system

Ossification in a muscle.

Cause:

The cause is usually trauma to a muscle followed by bleeding, inflammation and fibrosis. Deposition of bone-forming tissue in the muscle can result in calcification in the muscle producing this condition. The osteoblasts (bone forming cells) may originate from the injured periosteum adjacent to the injured muscle or could be by transformation of cells in the injured tissue. The ossified tissue, apart from restricting movement serves as a constant source of irritation to the surrounding soft tissue.

Signs and Symptoms:

The individual gives a history of fracture or trauma which is followed by reduced movement, pain and swelling in the local area. A hard mass may be felt in the injured region.

Risk factors:

The brachialis muscle is a common site for myositis ossificans. The incidence is higher after a supracondylar fracture and posterior dislocation of the elbow. Some believe that the risk is higher if a fractured part is mobilized too soon, too vigorously.

Caution and Recommendations to Therapists:

Do not forcibly mobilize joints especially the elbow, if there is restriction to extension. Consult physician regarding the cause of the restriction before embarking on mobilization techniques. Tenderness, signs of inflammation (swelling, increase in temperature etc.) in an injured muscle especially in the brachialis should be treated with great caution. Massage should be avoided in and around the area.

Notes: ───

Myositis ossificans is treated by immobilization and anti-inflammatory drugs. If no improvement is seen, surgery may be required.

Nephrotic syndrome   Renal system

A collection of symptoms that result from leakiness of the glomeruli to plasma protein.

Cause:

It can be a result of chronic glomerular disease. Diabetes mellitus, systemic lupus erythematosus are other disorders that result in increased permeability of the glomeruli.

Signs and Symptoms:

The loss of protein in the urine along with the retention of sodium and water causes extensive generalized edema. The loss of antibodies (immunoglobulins) makes the individual susceptible to infections. Loss of blood factors (also plasma proteins) that inhibit coagulation makes the person prone to thrombus formation. The increased level of lipids in the blood that also results, makes the individual prone to atherosclerosis. The blood pressure is elevated.

Risk factors:

See Cause.

Caution and Recommendations to Therapists:

A very light, soothing massage of short duration can be given. Do not try to reduce the edema that is present as it may overload the heart. Encourage client to be active and exercise as it can help reduce the chances of thrombus formation. These individuals are susceptible to infections. Avoid treating if harboring any infection.

Notes: ────────────────────────────────────

This condition is treated supportively. Diet restriction and antibiotics, diuretics and corticosteroids form part of the treatment regime.

Neurofibromatosis (NF, Von Recklinghausen's disease, Neurofibroma, Neurofibromata, Multiple neuroma, Neuromatosis)

Musculoskeletal, Integumentary, Nervous, Endocrine, Renal systems

An inherited disorder affecting many systems, characterized by formation of soft, multiple tumors along peripheral nerves.

Cause:

It is caused by defects in chromosome 17, or 21. It is inherited from an affected parent and there is 50% chance of the child inheriting the defective gene, regardless of sex. Since it is a dominant trait the disease is seen in an affected child even if one parent is normal. In 50% of cases, it is caused by a new mutation ie. a new defect in the chromosome. The symptoms are caused by abnormal multiplication of tissue - Schwann cells, that surround peripheral nerves.

Signs and Symptoms:

It is characterized by multiple, soft growths of varying sizes along the nerves. There may also be uniformly darkened, large, flat lesions on the skin. The skin lesions are known as cafe-au-lait spots. The symptoms usually appear in childhood or adolescence and may stop as the child matures. The growths may produce additional symptoms by compressing surrounding tissues. Compression of nerves inside the skull or spinal column can produce neurological problems like blindness, seizures, mental deficiency etc. In addition, other systems may be involved. Skeletal involvement can produce scoliosis, kyphosis and vertebral column defects. It can also affect the endocrine system resulting in hyper or hyposecretion of various glands. The kidney can also be affected leading to renal failure.

Risk factors:

See Cause

Caution and Recommendations to Therapists:

This is a genetic condition, and not infective, though the skin and tumors may look unsightly. It is important for the therapist to provide emotional support to the client who may be marginalized by society because of the appearance of the skin. A detailed history should be taken to assess the extent of the disease and massage treatment individualized accordingly. There is no danger of spreading the tumors by massage. Refer client to local support groups and for genetic counselling if in the reproductive age group (see Appendix IV for resources).

Notes: _____

Nutritional deficiencies - Vitamin A

Gastrointestinal system

The deficiency of Vitamin A which is one of the fat-soluble vitamins.

Cause:

It is usually caused by inadequate intake of food stuff high in this vitamin. High levels of vitamin A is present in liver, kidney, butter, milk, cream, cheese, fortified margarine, green leafy vegetables, eggyolk, yellow and orange fruits. Since this vitamin is fat soluble, deficiency states are also found in those who have difficulty in absorbing fats. Fat absorption is altered in people with liver disorders, malabsorption syndromes etc.

Signs and Symptoms:

Since vitamin A participates in the functioning of the receptors in the eye, as well as in the formation of epithelium and bone growth, symptoms are associated with these sites. The first symptom is night blindness - difficulty in seeing in dark places. Drying of the conjunctiva with thickened gray colored spots in the conjunctiva are other symptoms. Untreated, this can lead to blindness. The skin is dry and scaly. The hardening and drying of the mucous membranes makes them prone for infections.

Risk factors:

See Cause.

Caution and Recommendations to Therapists:

Encourage clients to eat green leafy vegetables and fruits along with adequate intake of dairy products. Those with problems in absorption may require Vitamin A in the form of injections. Advice clients on the harmful effects of excessive intake of vitamin supplements (see Hypervitaminosis).

Use oil liberally while massaging clients with dry skin. Refer clients complaining of night-blindness to a Physician.

Notes: ───

Recommended dietary allowance: 1,400IU(children); 4000-5000IU(adults); 6000IU(lactating women).

Nutritional deficiencies - Vitamin B

Gastrointestinal system

The deficiency of Vitamin B complex - a group of water-soluble vitamins.

Cause:

It usually results from inadequate intake or malabsorption of the vitamins.

Vitamin B1 - thiamine deficiency is seen in those whose staple diet is unenriched rice or wheat. Malnourishment, alcoholism and pregnancy are other conditions that can predispose to thiamine deficiency.

Vitamin B2 - riboflavin deficiency results when the intake of milk, meat, fish, green leafy vegetables are inadequate. Absorption of this vitamin is reduced in alcoholics and in those with prolonged diarrhea.

Niacin - another of the B complex vitamins, is seen in those whose diet lacks animal protein or whose staple food is corn.

Pyridoxine(B6) deficiency is usually a side effect of those taking drugs such as isoniazid (antituberculosis) which are pyridoxine antagonists.

Cobalamin - *vitamin B12* deficiency usually results in those with difficulty in absorption of Vitamin B12. Vitamin B12 requires a factor - called intrinsic factor that is secreted by the stomach, for proper absorption in the ileum. Those who lack this intrinsic factor, or those who have had surgery where the stomach or ileum has been removed can show signs of cobalamin deficiency.

Signs and Symptoms:

These vitamins are required for cell growth, bone formation and normal breakdown of food products.

Vitamin B1 deficiency - Beriberi, mainly affects the nervous system. Irritability, mental disturbances, gait abnormalities are some of the symptoms. It can also be a cause of edema. Abdominal pain, vomiting, convulsions are other symptoms. It also affects the cardiovascular system producing enlargement of the heart, rapid heart rate and cardiac failure.

Riboflavin deficiency produces cracking of the lips and corners of the mouth, sore throat, inflammation of the tongue.The skin appears dry and scaly. In children the growth may be slowed.

Niacin deficiency produces vague symptoms such as fatigue, loss of appetite, muscle weakness, weight loss, indigestion etc. In advanced stages (pellagra), the skin becomes darkened and scaly. The mouth, tongue and lips become sore. The central nervous system may be affected with confusion and other mental disturbances. It is also called the "3-D syndrome" - Dementia, Diarrhea and Dermatitis. Pyridoxine deficiency resembles that of niacin deficiency.

B12 deficiency affects the development of red blood cells and results in anemia. Anemia produced by B12 deficiency is known as Pernicious anemia. Associated symptoms include loss of weight, constipation, diarrhea, inflammation of the tongue and nervous disorders like spasticity of the muscles and gait abnormalities.

Risk factors:

See Cause.

Caution and Recommendation to Therapists:

Use oil liberally in those with dry scaly skin. Encourage clients to take a well balanced diet. While vitamin supplements do have a role to play, there is no substitute for a well balanced diet.

Notes: ──

Recommended daily requirement of Vitamin B complex:

Vitamin (men; women): B1 (1.4mg; 1.0mg); B2 (1.6mg; 1.2mg); Niacin (18mg; 13mg); B6 (2.2mg; 2.0mg); B12 (3mcg; 3mcg).

═══

Nutritional deficiencies - Vitamin C
(Scurvy)   Gastrointestinal system

A condition where there is a deficiency of ascorbic acid - vitamin C, a water-soluble vitamin.

Cause:

It is usually due to the deficient intake of vitamin C in the diet. Vitamin C is destroyed by overcooking and on overexposure to air. So deficiency may result if the cooking process destroys it.

Signs and Symptoms:

Since vitamin C is required for the production of collagen - a component of connective tissue that helps bind cells of teeth, bones and capillaries together, deficiency of it presents as abnormalities in these tissues. The capillaries become fragile and break easily. Small spots of bleeding under the skin are seen (see Appendix 1 figure 10). The person is anemic, with loss of appetite, limb and joint pain. The gums become swollen and bleed easily. Wounds take a longer time to heal. Irritability and depression are some of the psychological problems. This disease is potentially fatal.

Risk factors:

See Cause.

Caution and Recommendations to Therapists:

Encourage client to drink fresh orange juice. Advice client on the harm of taking too much vitamin C. Excess Vitamin C causes, vomiting, diarrhea and formation of stone in the kidney. Do not use excessive pressure as the client tends to bleed easily.

_____

Citrus fruits, tomatoes, cabbage, broccoli, spinach and berries are some of the food rich in vitamin C.

About 100-200mg of vitamin C is required per day. The vitamin has to be replenished every day as it cannot be stored.

===

Nutritional deficiencies - Vitamin D

(Rickets, Osteomalacia)   Gastrointestinal system

A condition due to the deficiency of Vitamin D - calciferol, a fat-soluble vitamin.

Cause:

Vitamin D can result from inadequate intake, malabsorption in the gut, or low exposure to sunlight. Rarely, it occurs as an inherited disorder where there is excessive loss of phosphates in the urine. Vitamin D being fat-soluble, is not absorbed in gastrointestinal disorders that affect fat absorption - liver disease, malabsorption syndrome, obstruction to the bile duct etc. Since vitamin D requires normal secretion of parathormone from the parathyroid gland, and is altered to its active form in the kidney and liver, diseases of parathyroid gland, liver or kidney can also result in deficiency states.

Signs and Symptoms:

Vitamin D is required for normal bone formation as it participates in the absorption and regulation of calcium and phosphorus and its lack present as bone deformities. Early symptoms are excessive sweating, restlessness and irritability. The bones become soft resulting in bow legs, knock knees, pigeon chest, enlargement of the wrist and ankles and thickening of the costochondral junction. These deformities can produce problems in walking, climbing stairs etc.

Risk factors:

Breast fed infants who do not have supplements are prone to this problem. It is more common in overcrowded urban areas.

Caution and Recommendations to Therapists:

The bones are prone to fracture easily. Only light pressure should be used while massaging these individuals. Encourage clients to increase intake of vitamin rich food stuff such as cod liver oil, herring, liver, egg yolk, and fortified milk. Exposure to the sun should also be encouraged.

Notes: ────────────────────────────────────

Injection of Vitamin D is required for those with deficiency due to malabsorption. Recommended dietary allowance: 400IU daily.

Nutritional deficiencies - Vitamin E

Gastrointestinal system

Deficiency of vitamin E - tocopherol, a fat-soluble vitamin.

Cause:

It is usually caused by malabsorption of fat from the gut as in malabsorption syndrome, liver disease, bile duct blockage etc. Vitamin E is required for normal metabolism of fatty acids and other lipids inside the cells. Rarely, low intake of vitamin E causes this problem. Diets rich in Vitamin E are vegetable oils, green leafy vegetables, nuts and legumes. Deficiency may also result in people whose diet includes high consumption of polyunsaturated fatty acids.

Signs and Symptoms:

Deficiency of vitamin E is difficult to recognize. It can present with edema, red raised skin lesions that slowly peels, or muscle weakness. In new born children it can present as anemia.

Risk factors:

See Cause.

Caution and Recommendations to Therapists:

Encourage client to take a well balanced diet.

Notes: ─────────────────────────────────────

Nutritional deficiencies - Vitamin K

Deficiency of Vitamin K, a fat-soluble vitamin - one of the components required for normal coagulation of blood.

Cause:

Vitamin K is normally produced by the organisms present in the intestines. Drugs such as antibiotics, that destroy these organisms in the gut can lead to vitamin K deficiency. The anticoagulant dicoumarol that is given to people with venous thrombosis, reduces thrombus formation by antagonizing vitamin K. Therefore, in a person on prolonged treatment with anticoagulants, vitamin K deficiency occurs. In those with difficulty in the digestion and absorption of fat, this deficiency may result. Liver disease, bile duct obstruction, malabsorption syndrome are some of the other conditions that can lead to such a state. Rarely, it may due to inadequate intake of vitamin K.

Signs and Symptoms:

The main symptom is a tendency to bleed easily and an increase in time for clotting to occur. The bleeding can be severe and fatal.

Risk factors:

See Cause.

Caution and Recommendations to Therapists:

A proper history is required from a client who is on anticoagulant therapy. Since there is a tendency to bleed, pressure can cause tiny bleeding spots under the skin (see Appendix I figure 10). A very gentle and light massage is all that should be attempted in such clients. Vitamin K deficiency can be treated very easily and it may be best to postpone a massage till adequate treatment has been taken. If the deficiency has resulted in a client on treatment for venous thrombosis, consult physician before scheduling a massage.

Notes: ————————————————————————————————————

Obesity   Gastrointestinal, Endocrine, Musculoskeletal systems

An increase in adipose tissue that imparts a health risk. It has been shown that weights exceeding 20% of the expected weight for that age, sex and height is a definite health risk.

Cause:

It is caused by intake of nutrients more than the expenditure or when the expenditure is less than the intake. Many factors influence the intake. There are feeding centers and satiety centers located in the hypothalamus which regulate the intake in accordance to the glucose/insulin levels in the blood. These centers also sense the distention of the stomach and the amount of body fat. In addition the centers are sensitive to catecholamine levels. This explains the weight loosing effect of the drug amphetamine. However, ultimately the cerebral cortex controls the eating behavior. Thus psychological, social and genetic factors have an effect on weight.

Obesity may be secondary to other diseases like Hypothyroidism, Cushing's disease and hypothalamic disorders, among others.

Signs and Symptoms:

Obesity is associated with an increase in the incidence of many diseases. The incidence of Diabetes mellitus is higher. This may be due to the resistance of tissues in obese individuals to insulin. The increased levels of cholesterol in the bile make these individuals prone for developing gallstones. The excess mechanical and physical stress on various body-systems result in disorders like osteoarthritis, sciatica, varicose veins, thromboembolism and hernias. Hypertension, atherosclerosis are also common increasing the risk of angina and stroke.

Risk factors:

See Cause.

Caution and Recommendations to Therapists:

Most obese individuals have a low self esteem so therapists have to be sensitive to the needs of these individuals. Excessive pressure may be needed to massage even the superficial muscles. Ensure that the massage table is sufficiently study. After a good rapport has been established, encourage client to loose weight by altering dietary intake, behavior modification and lifestyle.

Notes: ──

To be accurate, obesity is determined by measuring the thickness of the skin in various areas of the body like the skin over the triceps or below the scapula. In general, a deficit of 7700 kcal results in he loss of about 1kg fat.

Osteochondrosis (Osgood-Schlatter disease)
Musculoskeletal system

A painful, incomplete separation of the epiphysis of the tibial tubercle from the tibial shaft and/or tendinitis of the patellar tendon at its insertion to the tibial tubercle.

Cause:

Trauma to the area before the fusion of the tibial epiphysis before adulthood is the commonest cause. The trauma may be a single episode or repeated knee flexion against an unyielding quadriceps. It affects single or both knees.

Signs and Symptoms:

It presents as a constant ache, pain and tenderness below the patella which is worsened on climbing stairs, squatting or any activity involving flexion of knee. Signs of inflammation - heat, swelling and tenderness may be present.

Risk factors:

It is more common in active adolescent boys. Genetic factors are also associated.

Caution and Recommendations to Therapists:

Ice massage and rest are recommended in the initial stages. This condition used to be treated by immobilization for 6-8 weeks, but recently rehabilitative exercises are used. Stretching with ankle dorsiflexion and strengthening of leg muscles should be resorted to if weakness is found. Patellar support also helps. Use friction massage around the knee to stretch collagen fibres and reduce adhesions.

Notes:

Osteogenesis Imperfecta (Brittle bones, Fragilitas ossium)

Musculoskeletal system

An inherited disorder that affects the development of connective tissue and bones.

Cause:

It is transmitted to a child from an affected parent, regardless of sex, usually as a dominant trait ie. presenting as a disease even if both parents are not affected.

Signs and Symptoms:

It is characterized by thin and underdeveloped bones that are very prone to fracture with the most trivial trauma. In a child, the face appears triangular due to the soft and prominent forehead. The person is short in stature, with thin skin, blue sclera, hypotonic muscles and loose-jointedness.

Risk factors:

See Cause.

Caution and Recommendations to Therapists:

Do not massage a client with this condition as they are very prone to fractures.

Notes:

Osteomyelitis

(osteo - bone, myelo - bone marrow)

A bone infection.

Cause:

It can be caused iatrogenically - ie. as a complication after surgical or other treatment. Infection can also be spread to the bone through the blood from another infected site. Direct contamination as in gun shot wound, trauma, open fracture, or by spreading from an adjacent infection are other causes. Infection persisting beyond 6-8 weeks is considered to be chronic osteomyelitis. This is usually due to inadequately treated acute osteomyelitis.

Signs and Symptoms:

Symptoms vary according to whether it is acute or chronic. In acute osteomyelitis, the tibia, femur, humerus or radius are affected more frequently. The client has fever along with pain, redness and swelling over the bone. In chronic osteomyelitis, there may be shortening or lengthening of the limb due to overgrowth caused by increased blood flow to the area. If the joints are affected, deformity, stiffening and dislocation may occur.

Risk factors:

Open fracture, gunshot wounds, extensive tissue injury with contamination, complication of surgery involving bones and joints are all risk factors. Osteomyelitis is more common in those below 20 years of age.

Caution and Recommendations to Therapists:

In clients with unhealed or recently healed wounds keep the area covered with bandage and avoid local massage. In clients who have been healed, the aim is to help restore the strength of muscles around the affected area and improve movement in stiff joints if not ankylosed. Use friction strokes and vibration around adherent scars. Olive oil can be used to help soften the fibrous tissue. If there are signs of inflammation or pus discharge from an old scar it indicates reinfection. Stop treatment and refer to physician.

Notes:

Clients are treated with long term antibiotics and surgery to remove dead tissue or foreign bodies like metal plates etc.

Osteoporosis

A disorder where the bone resorption is greater than bone formation.

Cause:

It occurs as part of the aging process and begins around the age of 25. It can also result from endocrine disorders or malignancy. In this condition both the organic as well as the mineral content of bone is reduced.

Signs and Symptoms:

The bone is fragile and brittle and fractures easily with minimal stress. Bone pain and stress fractures are usually the first symptoms.

Risk factors:

Osteoporosis is more common in post menopausal women. The progress is also faster in women as compared to men. Reduced sex hormone levels in the blood have been shown to speed up resorption of bone. Caucasians are affected more often. Poor nutrition, decrease in intestinal absorption of calcium and a sedentary lifestyle are some of the predisposing factors. It may also be caused by excessive exercise. Osteoporosis is also common in people with endocrine disorders such as hyperthyroidism, hyperparathyroidism, Cushing's syndrome, diabetes mellitus and with prolonged use of corticosteroids. Aluminium containing antacids that increase calcium excretion and anticonvulsants are some of the drugs that increase the risk of osteoporosis.

Cigarette smoking, high protein diet, alcoholism and family history of osteoporosis are other known risk factors. Prolonged immobilization of a limb increases resorption of bone and osteoporosis. It is also seen in people with rheumatoid arthritis.

Caution and Recommendations to Therapists:

Encourage clients to exercise. Use gentle massage avoiding undue pressure over bones in all postmenopausal and geriatric clients.

Notes:

Oseoporosis is detected by gauging the density of bones. It is best treated by elimination of risk factors and adequate dietary intake of calcium. Postmenopausal women are treated with estrogen therapy to slow down the process. However, estrogen therapy may predispose to some forms of uterine cancer.

The normal requirement of calcium in an adult is 800mg per day. The requirement is more during pregnancy and nursing. Good calcium supplements are available in the form of calcium gluconate or calcium citrate.

Ovarian cysts

Fluid filled cavities in the ovary.

Cause:

Ovarian cysts are usually formed by the persistence of follicles that mature during every menstrual cycle. The cysts may be single or multiple.

Signs and Symptoms:

It is usually asymptomatic. In some, a dull aching pain may be felt on the affected side. If the cyst gets twisted or ruptures, the person will have severe abdominal pain. Since the ovaries also secrete the hormones that are responsible for the menstrual cycle, the cycles may be irregular. In those with multiple cysts, infertility is common.

Risk factors:

It is common in women between puberty and menopause.

Caution and Recommendations to Therapists:

Do not massage the abdomen if a client has been diagnosed with a cyst. Pressure on the cyst can rupture it and cause severe pain in the individual.

Notes:

Ovarian cysts usually disappear spontaneously and do not require treatment. In some, it is treated with hormones like progesterone which cause the cysts to regress. Surgery may be done for abnormally large cysts, or those which show malignant changes.

Paget's disease (Osteitis Deformans)

A progressive metabolic disease of bone.

Cause:

The cause is unknown. It may be caused by a virus that can absorb bone. It is theorized that previous viral infections like mumps may cause a dormant skeletal infection that later presents as Paget's disease.

Signs and Symptoms:

The disease begins slowly and progresses over many years. There is an imbalance in the destruction, resorption and regrowth of bone. As a result the affected bone is replaced by fibrous tissue which gives the bone a rough and pitted outer surface. The symptoms depend on the area affected. A large proportion of people are asymptomatic. Lesions of the skull could result in headaches, ringing of the ears, dizziness and hearing loss. If the spine is affected, kyphosis may occur. If the long bones of the legs are affected, bow legs or knock knees may be seen. The gait may be waddling as a result. Pathological fractures may occur with the slightest injury as the disease makes the bones fragile and weak. Bone pain may be present in the affected area.

Risk factors:

It affects people over the age of 40 and more men are affected than women.

Caution and Recommendations to Therapists:

These clients are likely to be on pain killers and antiinflammatory drugs. Hence the feedback from the clients may be inadequate during massage. Massage gives symptomatic relief only. Do not use excessive pressure as they are prone for pathological fractures.

Notes:

It is treated with drugs like calcitonin to decrease bone resorption and pain killers. Paget's disease may be associated with osteogenic sarcoma.

Pancreatitis

An inflammation of the pancreas.

Cause:

The common causes are disease of the bile ducts and alcoholism. The bile duct disease causes back flow of bile into the pancreas. This occurs as the secretions of the pancreas and the bile flow into the duodenum through a common opening. The reflux of the bile activates the protein and fat digesting enzymes of the pancreas causing autodigestion of the pancreas and surrounding tissue. Alcohol is a direct stimulant of pancreatic secretion. The increased secretion along with bile reflux may be the cause of pancreatitis in alcoholics.

Signs and Symptoms:

Acute onset of pancreatitis typically occurs after intake of a heavy, fatty meal and alcohol. There is severe pain radiating to the back. The intensity of pain increases on lying down and is reduced on bending forward. There is abdominal distention accompanied by low grade fever, cold and sweaty palms. If the endocrine part of the pancreas is also damaged, diabetes mellitus results.

In chronic pancreatitis, as seen in alcoholics, the pancreas is slowly destroyed with reduced secretion of enzymes. The symptoms are that of malabsorption syndrome in this case. Recurrent and persistent pain localized to the upper left quadrant of the abdomen and below the sternum is present.

Risk factors:

Alcohol intake, high fatty diet, drugs such as corticosteroids, certain diuretics and antibiotics can predispose to pancreatitis.

Caution and Recommendations to Therapists:

Acute pancreatitis is a medical emergency and could be fatal. Avoid abdominal massage in those with chronic pancreatitis. Encourage client to take a low fat diet. Refer to local support groups if an alcoholic. Refer to Appendix IV for resources.

Notes: ————————————————————————————————

Parkinson's disease (Shaking palsy, Paralysis Agitans, Parkinsonism)

Nervous system

A chronic, progressive disorder affecting the motor system.

Cause:

It is produced by a deficiency of the neurotransmitter dopamine in the basal ganglia of the brain. It may also be due to overactivity of acetylcholine in the same area. Since this area participates in muscle coordination and plays an inhibitory part in motor function, the symptoms are typically related to the motor system.

Signs and Symptoms:

The symptoms may begin slowly and the disease may progress at different rates in each individual. There is muscle rigidity (increased tone on passively stretching a muscle), typically called lead pipe rigidity as the rigidity is present throughout the range of motion. The rigidity results in alterations in posture and gait. The person is bent forward from the hips and stands with the knees and hips flexed. The head is also flexed. Tremors at rest - typically a pill rolling movement of the fingers are present. The tremor is exaggerated when stressed and is reduced on performing a purposeful movement or during sleep.

The gait is abnormal and is shuffling or hurrying in type. On walking, the person seems to be trying to catch his/her center of gravity with a tendency to walk faster and faster with shorter steps. The natural swinging of the arm is absent with walking. The face is mask-like - lacking in expression and the tone of the voice is monotonous. The general coordination is difficult and there is difficulty in eating, swallowing, speaking and writing. However, the intellect is normal. There is no sensory loss but the person may suffer from cramps and aches. There may be sudden sensations of heat, and increased sweating in certain areas of the body. Constipation and loss of bladder control is also common.These individuals are prone to depression.

Risk factors:

It affects men more commonly. It occurs more frequently between the age of 50-60. Rarely, Parkinsonism is seen after carbon monoxide poisoning, cerebro vascular accidents (stroke), tumors in the region of the basal ganglia, drug treatment for schizophrenia and other psychiatric disorders.

Caution and Recommendations to Therapists:

The aim of treatment is to reduce the rigidity and maintain bowel movements. A full body relaxation massage definitely reduces the symptoms, though temporarily. Use gentle, slow to moderate speed, repetitive, rhythmic strokes starting with the back - the least rigid area, before moving on to the shoulder, neck and upper limbs. Use effleurage and light to moderate pressure friction. Passively move all joints after the massage - but do not use force. Massage in a prone position helps to counteract the flexing effect of the disease - but elderly clients may feel uncomfortable in this position. Abdominal massage helps relieve constipation in these individuals. Use clockwise movements - along the direction of movement in the colon. Special vibration techniques called "pushing" along with effleurage have been found to be useful.

The total duration of the massage should be short lasting for about half an hour with equal time spent in all areas. Some Massage Therapists have found treatment schedules that include a total of 15 sessions, two to three times per week followed by a break for one to two months with repetition of the same sequence, to be beneficial to the client. (See Appendix IV for resources.)

Encourage the clients to be as active as possible. Refer the client to local support groups.

Notes: ───

The disease is progressive and chronic and treatment - at present, is to slow down or stop the progress of the disease. These clients are treated with levo-dopa - a drug which increases the level of dopamine in the brain. Anticholinergics that reduce acetyl choline levels in the area are also used. In some individuals surgery may be resorted to. Research is underway to explore the possibilities of transplant. Alternative therapy include water exercises like swimming, yoga, tai chi and aerobic exercises within tolerable levels. To reduce constipation high fibre diet is recommended.

═══

Paronychia

Integumentary system

An acute or chronic infection of the nail folds on the finger.

Cause:

It is usually caused by the bacteria Staphylococcus aureus.

Signs and Symptoms:

The nail fold appears swollen and tender and pus may be expressed after gentle pressure in acute lesions. In chronic lesions pain and swelling may be mild.

Risk factors:

It is common in individuals whose fingers are subjected to repeated immersion in water or food stuffs. It may be a super infection of eczema affecting the area.

Caution and Recommendations to Therapists:

Avoid local area while massaging. To prevent the occurrence of paronychia, avoid prolonged immersion of hands and feet in water. Carefully dry nail folds after washing.

Notes: ───

═══

Pediculosis (Lice)   Integumentary system

An infestation with lice - wingless insects that feed on human and animal blood.

Cause:

Three types of lice infect man - body lice (pediculus humanus corporis), pubic lice (pediculus pubis or crabs) and head lice (pediculus humanus capitis). The lice go through different stages - egg (nit) laid along the hair shaft, moult stage and adult stage. The life span of a louse is between 30 to 50 days. An adult lice is as big as a pinhead, light grey or brown in color.

The body lice can survive for 10 to 14 days in beddings, seams of clothes etc., unlike the head lice which dies within a day outside the body. The pubic lice can live away from the body for up to two days.

Signs and Symptoms:

The client, if affected with body lice will complain of itching especially in the shoulder, back and buttock area. Itchy, reddened and raised areas may be seen on the body.

In head lice, nits may be found in the hair. Nits are pearl-gray or brown, oval structures found on the hair shaft close to the scalp. The scalp may appear red and raw due to scratching. Rarely, an adult louse may be sighted.

Risk factors:

Living in a crowded environment in contact with an infected individual places a person at risk.

Caution and Recommendations to Therapists:

Although no serious complications result from infestation with lice, it is annoying to have this infestation. Also, the social stigma attached to lice infestation can ruin the prospects of a clinic if a client contracts lice after a visit. Lice spreads from close contact with an infested person. Massage is contraindicated.

In body lice infestation, since the lice can survive without the host for a long time, the bedding and linen should be washed in boiling water and steam pressed or dry cleaned if a client has been massaged inadvertently. Clothes can also be disinfected by keeping them in air tight bags for two weeks or more. Special shampoos and body lotions with malathion or pyrethrum are available. Mattresses and upholstery should be vacuumed and disinfected.

Similar treatment is given for pubic and head lice infestations. Nits from hair can also be removed using a fine toothed comb. If a shampoo is used, the treatment should be repeated after a week to kill newly hatched lice.

Notes: —————————————————————————————————————

Pelvic Inflammatory Disease (PID)

Reproductive system

Any inflammation of the organs in the female pelvis. It includes inflammation of the fallopian tubes, ovaries, uterus and supporting tissues.

Cause:

It is usually caused by bacteria (Chlamydia) living in the vagina, or which has been transmitted sexually.

Signs and Symptoms:

Fever, lower abdominal pain and tenderness, pain on having intercourse and white discharge from the vagina are the common symptoms.

Risk factors:

It is more common in women between 16-24 with multiple sexual partners. The risk is increased with the use of intrauterine devices for contraception.

Caution and Recommendations to Therapists:

Encourage client to take the full course of the prescribed antibiotics. Educate the client that sexual partners may also have to be treated to prevent reinfection. Avoid abdominal area while massaging the client. The client may feel more comfortable in a position with the head and knee raised with pillows. There is no scope for the transmission of infection as it is sexually transmitted. Ask client to keep underclothes on during massage. The standard precautions for any infection should be taken (see appendix II).

Notes: ──

A full course of antibiotics for 14 days is required to control the disease. If inadequately treated, adhesions can form between the organs in the pelvis, or the tubes may become blocked leading to complications such as infertility, ectopic pregnancy, or abscesses in the pelvis.

Peptic ulcer   Gastrointestinal system

Ulcers in the mucosa of the esophagus, stomach (gastric), duodenum or jejunum.

Cause:

The commonest cause is infection of the mucosa with Helicobacter Pylori (Campylobacter pylori). Use of non steroidal anti-inflammatory drugs and other conditions that increase the acid secretion of the stomach and/or breakdown the mucosal barrier that prevents the erosion of the stomach wall by the acid, cause peptic ulcer.

Signs and Symptoms:

It varies with the location of the ulcer. In gastric ulcer, there is indigestion and heartburn. The person may loose weight. There may be associated bleeding from the stomach resulting in blood in vomitus or dark tarry stools (melena).

In duodenal ulcer, the pain produced is similar to that of gastric ulcer but is relieved by food. However, it comes on about two hours after ingestion of food. The picture may be complicated by formation of stricture in the intestinal end of the stomach - pyloric stenosis.

Risk factors:

Ingestion of alcohol, smoking, intake of steroids or non-steroidal anti inflammatory drugs in an empty stomach are all risk factors. It affects men more than women. Gastric ulcers are more common between fifty and sixty years of age. Stress and anxiety contribute to the formation of ulcers as they reduce the secretion of mucus in the walls of the duodenum. This mucus production, which is inhibited by sympathetic stimulation, serves to protect the stomach lining.

Caution and Recommendations to Therapists:

Avoid massage to the upper abdominal area. Massage helps reduce stress - a predisposing factor to ulcers. Encourage clients to take the full course of antibiotics and avoid alcohol and to stop smoking if a smoker.

Notes: ───

Antibiotics are given to combat the bacterial infection. Other medical or surgical measures are taken to decrease acid secretion in the stomach.

Periodontitis

An inflammation of the oral mucosa around the teeth.

Cause:

Signs and Symptoms:

Risk factors: same as Gingivitis

Caution and Recommendations to Therapists:

Notes: ───

Peripheral Neuritis (Multiple Neuritis, Peripheral Neuropathy, Polyneuritis)

Nervous system

A degenerative disorder of peripheral nerves especially those supplying the distal parts of the limbs (fingers and toes).

Cause:

It is a non-inflammatory degeneration of the sensory and motor nerves to the hand and toes. Many conditions have been associated with peripheral neuritis (see risk factors).

Signs and Symptoms:

The symptoms appear slowly, with atrophy and flaccid paralysis of the small muscles of the hand and feet. The sensation is also diminished with the vibratory sense being affected first. Footdrop may be present. The muscles may be tender and hypersensitive to touch and pressure. There may be decreased sweating and the skin appears red and glossy.

Risk factors:

It is more common in men between the ages of 30-50. Chronic alcoholism, lead poisoning, diabetes mellitus, gout, rheumatoid arthritis, Systemic Lupus Erythematous,vitamin deficiencies, excessive intake of sulphur containing drugs like sulphonamides have all been implicated. It has also been associated with infections like tuberculosis, diphtheria, meningitis, mumps and Guillain-Barre syndrome.

Caution and Recommendations to Therapists:

The aim is to increase the tone, prevent contractures and joint stiffness and to relieve pain if present. Care should be taken to avoid undue pressure as the sensations are diminished. Perform range of motion exercises to all the joints of the hand, but do not use force to increase the range. Use lymphatic drainage techniques to reduce edema if present. Use strokes that are directed from distal to proximal areas. Look for pressure ulcers - especially if the client is wearing splints or braces. Avoid areas of ulcers and give a wide margin around the area. Enriched oils (with high Vitamin A or Vitamin E content) can be used while massaging the affected areas.

Notes:

Although the treatment is supportive, the cause of the neuritis has to be established. High intake of vitamins especially vitamin B12 is required.

Peritonitis

An inflammation of the membrane (peritoneum) that lines the abdominal cavity and covers the organs in the abdomen.

Cause:

It can be caused by bacteria or by chemical irritation. Any condition that exposes the peritoneum to the contents of the intestine can cause this. Chemical irritation most often occurs after abdominal surgery.

Signs and Symptoms:

Pain and tenderness are the common symptoms. The pain is increased on moving the abdomen and the person lies still breathing shallowly. The abdominal muscles go into a spasm and become boardlike. There are signs of dehydration as the inflammation of the peritoneum causes fluid to ooze into the abdominal cavity. The movements of the intestines are reflexly stopped.

Risk factors:

Peptic ulcer that has perforated, ruptured appendix or bowel, inflamed gall bladder, abdominal trauma and wounds can predispose to peritonitis.

Caution and Recommendations to Therapists:

Usually, the client will be too sick to be massaged. Gentle and soothing massage with minimal movement of the client, avoiding the abdomen, can be given in a hospital setting to reduce stress and pain, after clearance from a physician.

Notes:

The treatment is supportive. Fluid and electrolyte balance is maintained. Antibiotics are given to combat infection and pain killers to reduce the pain.

Pheochromocytoma

A tumor of the adrenal medulla that secretes excess adrenaline and noradrenaline.

Cause:

The cause of the tumor is not known. It may be due to defective genes transmitted from the parent.

Signs and Symptoms:

The adrenal medulla secretes adrenaline and noradrenaline - which are also secreted as neurotransmitters by the sympathetic nervous system. Hence the symptoms resemble that of hyperactivity of the sympathetic nervous system - fight or flight reaction. The person has persistent increase in blood pressure. The heart rate is rapid. Excessive sweating, headache, flushed and warm skin, anxiety, nervousness and rapid respiration are some of the symptoms. The person also has dizziness on changing posture (postural hypotension). The symptoms persist or come on suddenly many times a day. The symptoms may be precipitated by exercise, laughing, urination, or any type of stress.

Risk factors:

See Cause.

Caution and Recommendations to Therapists:

Do not massage an individual before treatment. If necessary before treatment, massage should be undertaken only after physician's approval. Although massage helps reduce stress, palpation of the abdomen or lower back can bring on an attack of symptoms by direct stimulation of the tumor. These individuals are prone for postural hypotension and it should be ensured that changes in posture like getting off the table are done slowly and with support.

Notes: ───

It is treated by removing the tumor surgically.

Pityriasis Rosea   Integumentary system

An inflammatory skin disorder.

Cause:

The cause is unknown. It may be of viral origin and close contact with an infected individual may spread this condition.

Signs and Symptoms:

It appears as a single macule or papule surrounded by redness in the neck or trunk.

As it spreads the central area clears. The lesion fades in 2-10 days while a fresh crop begins to appear. The lesions disappear in 6-8 weeks. Some itching may be present.

Risk factors:

It is common in spring and fall seasons. The incidence is higher in young adults.

Caution and Recommendations to Therapists:

Do not massage the local area as it may be contagious.

The immunity may be suppressed if the client is on oral corticosteroids. Ensure that you do not have any mild form of infection while treating these clients as it may present more seriously if spread to these immunocompromised individuals. Wash hands thoroughly and disinfect linen and bed after massage treatment to clients with this condition.

Notes: _____

Plantar fasciitis
Musculoskeletal system

Inflammation of the plantar fascia and the surrounding structures.

Cause:

It is caused by excessive stress on the foot especially near the attachment of the fascia to the calcaneus bone. The stress causes calcium deposit in the site thus forming a spur.

Signs and Symptoms:

The person complains of pain in the heel which is made worse on climbing stairs,

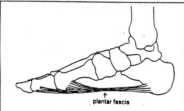
plantar fascia

walking or running. The pain is relieved by rest. There is tenderness near the attachment of the fascia to the calcaneus, medial aspect of the foot and in the abductor hallucis muscle. The pain is increased on stretching the plantar fascia by dorsiflexion. There is no loss of sensation. The plantar surface of the foot may be red and swollen.

Risk factors:

It is more common in individuals with high arched foot, and those over the age of 40. In the younger age group it can occur in those who are active in sports. People who are in occupations that involve prolonged standing or walking are also prone.

Caution and Recommendations to Therapists:

Ice massage and rest is used initially. In the subacute or chronic stage, friction massage at the origin of the calcaneus is given to reduce adhesions. Mobilize the joints of the foot, to reduce stiffness. Lymphatic massage and drainage techniques can be used in the leg and ankle. The muscles of the leg should be massaged thoroughly to increase circulation and reduce spasm and trigger points. Remedial exercises to stretch the gastrocnemius and the plantar fascia should also be done. The client may be on anti-inflammatory drugs, and this may prevent them from giving a proper feedback regarding pressure and otherwise painful techniques.

Treatments lasting for half an hour, at a frequency of two to three times a week are recommended.

Notes: ───

Pleural effusion

Respiratory system

Denotes an excess of fluid in the pleural space.

Cause:

The cause is similar to that of edema. When the pressure in the lung capillaries increase or when the osmotic pressure in the blood decreases, fluid from the blood tends to collect in spaces outside the blood vessels of which the pleural space is one. Such a situation can be produced in heart failure, liver disease, reduced protein in the blood as in malnutrition or kidney failure. Pleural effusion can also be produced when the capillaries become more permeable (leaky) as in inflammatory conditions, lung infections like tuberculosis, lung cancer or trauma to the chest.

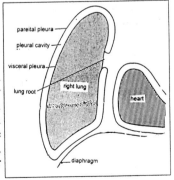

Signs and Symptoms:

Difficulty in breathing is present. The movement of the chest wall is decreased on the side of collection of fluid. There may be chest pain which is increased on movements produced by breathing. If there is pus in the pleural cavity (empyema) there may be associated fever and weakness. Sometimes the fluid in the pleural cavity may be bloody as in lung cancers or trauma (hemothorax). Rarely, the fluid may be lymph (chylothorax).

Risk factors:

It may be seen in individuals with Systemic Lupus Erythematosus (SLE) and Rheumatoid Arthritis.

Caution and Recommendations to Therapists:

Consult physician regarding cause of effusion. If due to infection do not massage till treated completely. If due to tuberculosis follow precautions given under tuberculosis. The aim is to help with the absorption of fluid, prevent adhesions, prevent permanent changes in posture and help with the ventilation. Avoid areas of drainage tube if it is in place. These clients have a tendency to develop scoliosis. The shoulder is lower and the hip higher on the affected side as compared to the normal side, so the postural muscles should be addressed while massaging. The treatments should be short - not more than fifteen minutes with more time spent to massage the arms, shoulder girdles and back. In chronic pleural effusion, massage with the client lying on the side with the normal side on the table helps to expand the affected lung. Ask client to push against your hand which is placed on the affected side, while breathing in. Deep breathing exercises are also helpful. Work in conjunction with a physiotherapist.

Notes: ————————————————————————————

If the fluid is excessive, it is treated in the hospital setting by drainage with a tube in the pleural cavity. If caused by infection antibiotics are also administered

Pleural space is the space between the lungs and the thoracic wall. It is lined by a thin membrane called pleura.

Pleurisy (Pleuritis)   Respiratory system

An inflammation of the pleura.

Cause:

Pleurisy develops as a complication of pneumonia, tuberculosis, Systemic Lupus

Erythematosus, cancer or trauma to the chest. It is caused by bacterial infection.

Signs and Symptoms:

It presents as an intense, sharp stabbing pain over the chest on breathing deeply. There will be difficulty in breathing. Fever is present and respiration is shallow and rapid. The client leans to the affected side to avoid pain. A dry cough may be present.

Risk factors:

See Cause.

Caution and Recommendations to Therapists:

Encourage client to breath deeply. Since it may be due to bacterial infection, massage should not be done until the cause has been identified. If due to other causes, a full body relaxation massage may be done with focus on the shoulder, back and arms. Encourage client to take bed rest.

Notes: ⎯⎯⎯⎯⎯⎯⎯⎯⎯⎯⎯⎯⎯⎯⎯⎯⎯⎯⎯⎯⎯⎯⎯⎯⎯⎯⎯⎯⎯

Pleura is the lining around the lungs and inside of the thoracic wall.

Pneumoconiosis - Asbestosis

Respiratory system

A progressive disease that produces diffuse fibrosis in the lung. One of the spectrum of diseases called pneumoconiosis that are a result of airborne pollutants that damage the lung.

Cause:

It is caused by inhalation of asbestos fibers. The defence reaction of the body to the inhaled fibres causes thickening of the pleura, and diffuse fibrosis of lungs.

Signs and Symptoms:

The individual has difficulty in breathing and has a dry cough. In advanced cases there is chest pain and recurrent respiratory infection.

Risk factors:

Workers involved in asbestos mines and mills, construction industry workers where asbestos is used for prefabrication, fireproofing and textile industries are more prone. Asbestos is also used in paints, plastics, brake and clutch linings. Families of asbestos workers are also prone as a result of asbestos fibres shaken off the clothings of the worker. Others are also at risk through inhalation of asbestos fibres from the waste piles of neighboring asbestos plants.

Caution and Recommendations to Therapists:

These clients are prone to respiratory infections. Schedule them at a time when they are unlikely to be exposed to other clients who may have respiratory infection. Do not massage them when you have a respiratory infection. There is a high incidence of tuberculosis in people with silicosis. Ensure that it is not so with the client you are treating. Encourage client to stop smoking, if smoker, as it speeds up the progress of the disease.

Do a whole body relaxation massage using hacking, clapping and vibration strokes over the chest. The latter helps to drain secretions better. Steam inhalation before start of treatment may be beneficial. Keep room at higher humidity and warmth.

Notes: ————————————————————————————————

Pneumoconiosis - Berylliosis (Beryllium poisoning, Beryllium disease)

Respiratory, Cardiovascular, Renal, Gastrointestinal, Integumentary systems

One of the spectrum of diseases called pneumoconiosis that are a result of airborne pollutants that damage the lung. It is a progressive disease that predominantly affects the lungs.

Cause:

It is caused by inhalation of beryllium dusts, fumes, and mists. Beryllium may also be absorbed through the skin. The mechanism by which it produces the effects is not known.

Signs and Symptoms:

If absorbed through the skin, beryllium produces itching and a rash and later an ulcer at the site. If inhaled, it produces swelling and ulceration of the mucosa of the nose. It may lead to perforation of the nasal septum. It may also be associated with a dry cough, pain below the sternum and difficulty in breathing. It may progress to right heart failure due to the increased resistance in the lungs to blood flow. Enlargement of the liver and spleen may also result.

Risk factors:

Beryllium alloy workers, cathode ray tube makers (cathode ray tube is used in television/computer monitors), gas mantle makers, missile technicians, nuclear reactor workers are all at risk. Families of beryllium workers exposed to it by dust shaken off the clothes of workers, individuals exposed to it through neighboring plants are also at risk.

Caution and Recommendations to Therapists:

Similar to Pneumoconiosis - Asbestosis.

Notes: _____

Pneumoconiosis - Coal Worker's
(Black lung disease, Coal miner's disease, Miner's asthma, Anthracosis, Anthracosilicosis)

Respiratory system

A progressive disease that produces nodules and fibrosis in the lung. One of the spectrum of diseases called pneumoconiosis that are a result of airborne pollutants that damage the lung.

Cause:

Chronic inhalation of coal dust - especially particles that are smaller than 5 microns in diameter. The body's defense mechanism in the form of macrophages engulf the coal dust, but are unable to process it. The macrophages die with release of enzymes into the surrounding tissue which produce a local inflammatory reaction that heals by fibrosis. This in turn affects the lung structure and function.

Signs and Symptoms:

It begins asymptomatically. Depending on the duration and intensity of exposure, presence of silica in addition to the coal dust, and the susceptibility of the individual, the symptoms progress to difficulty in breathing, fatigue, cough with black sputum and recurrent respiratory tract infection.

Risk factors:

Smoking speeds up the progress of the disease. Coal miners or others working with coal are susceptible.

Caution and Recommendations to Therapists:

Similar to Pneumoconiosis - Asbestosis

Notes: ————————————————————————————————

Pneumoconiosis - Silicosis

Respiratory system

A progressive disease that produces nodules and fibrosis in the lung. One of the spectrum of diseases called pneumoconiosis that are a result of airborne pollutants that damage the lung.

Cause:

It is caused by chronic inhalation and deposition of crystals of silica dust in the lungs. The body's defense mechanism in the form of macrophages engulf the silica but are unable to process it. The macrophages die with release of enzymes into the surrounding tissue which produce a local inflammatory reaction that heals by fibrosis. This in turn affects lung function.

Signs and Symptoms:

Initially this condition is asymptomatic. Later, there is difficulty in breathing, dry cough, chest pain and recurrent respiratory infection. There is a high incidence of tuberculosis in these individuals.

Risk factors:

Individuals working in industries or areas which are a source of silica such as ceramic (flint) manufacturers, cement, building materials like sandstone are prone. Silica is found in paints, porcelain, scouring soaps, wood fillers, mines of gold, coal, lead, zinc or iron. Foundry workers, boiler scalers and stone cutters are others exposed to silica dust.

Caution and Recommendations to Therapists:

Similar to Pneumoconiosis - Asbestosis.

Notes: ────────────────────────────────

Pneumonia Respiratory system

An acute infection of the lung tissue that can affect the exchange of gas.

Cause:

Pneumonia could be due to virus (chicken pox, measles, influenza), bacteria (streptococcus, staphylococcus), fungus, protozoa, mycobacteria, mycoplasma or rickettsia. The pneumonia may affect the bronchus and alveoli - broncho-pneumonia; affect part of a lobe - lobular pneumonia; or an entire lobe - lobar pneumonia. The infection produces inflammation in the lung with increased blood flow and fluid moving into the alveoli. Slowly, this is resolved by reabsorption of fluid into the blood and by expulsion as sputum.

Signs and Symptoms:

Cough with sputum, chest pain that increases with the movement of the chest accompanied by fever and chills are classical symptoms. The breathing may be noisy and difficult.

Risk factors:

Individuals with chronic illness such as cancer, asthma, other chronic obstructive pulmonary diseases, bronchiectasis and cystic fibrosis are prone. Smoking, malnutrition, alcoholism are other risk factors. Inhalation of toxic chemicals that damage the lung, naso-gastric tubes, tracheostomies, thoracic or abdominal surgery, coma, immune deficiency, immunosuppressive treatment also predispose to this condition. Individuals on antibiotics that kill the normal respiratory flora can put an individual at risk.

Caution and Recommendations to Therapists:

Do not massage in the acute stage. During recovery, massage may be given with the client in a half lying position with the upper body propped up with pillows. Ask client to breathe deeply while offering mild resistance to the expansion of the chest by placing your hand flat on the side of the chest. This helps to re-expand the lung tissue. Tapotement over the chest helps drain secretions. Massage the muscles of posture to increase tone and blood flow as Pneumonia tends to cause scoliosis. Passively move joints and massage the lower limbs vigorously to prevent disuse atrophy of muscles from the prolonged bed rest. Ensure that you do not come in contact with the respiratory secretions. Place tissues used by client in a leak proof bag before disposal.

Notes: ———

Pneumothorax Respiratory System

A condition where there is accumulation of air in the pleural space.

Cause:

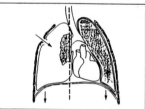

It may be due to abnormalities of the lung structure. In some individuals the lung tissue is weak and tends to give way to the pressure inside the lungs. There is escape of air into the pleural space as a result. This may happen in tuberculosis and emphysema. Trauma to the chest is another cause. Some times the opening is such that it allows air to enter but not leave the pleural cavity. This leads to tension pneumothorax and requires immediate assistance.

Signs and Symptoms:

The symptoms are produced by the pressure of the air in the pleura on the lung tissue and blood vessels. There is sudden, sharp pain that increases on movements produced by breathing. The chest wall moves unequally on both sides. Difficulty in breathing is experienced.

Risk factors:

Emphysema and tuberculosis increase the risk. Rarely there is a family history.

Caution and Recommendations to Therapists:

Consult physician. Do not massage unless cleared by physician.

Notes: ⎯⎯⎯⎯⎯⎯⎯⎯⎯⎯⎯⎯⎯⎯⎯⎯⎯⎯⎯⎯⎯⎯

Pleural space is the space between the lung and the thoracic cavity. It is lined by a thin membrane called pleura and has small quantities of fluid which reduce friction while breathing.

Wide bore needle may be used to drain out the excessive air in a hospital setting. It is treated with bed rest. Tension Pneumothorax is a surgical emergency.

Poliomyelitis (Polio, Infantile paralysis)

Nervous system

An acute viral infection which causes paralysis.

Cause:

It is caused by the polio virus which are of many types. The virus is transmitted from person to person by direct contact with infected saliva, droplets from the nose and throat or faeco-oral contamination. The incubation period is 5 - 35 days. The virus enters the body through the gut, multiplying in the pharynx and then spreading to the lymph nodes and blood. The virus specifically affects the neurons in the anterior horn - the motor neurons that supply muscles.

Signs and Symptoms:

Ninety-five percent of infections do not produce any signs and symptoms. Four to eight percent of cases subside after sore throat, vomiting and fever lasting for 2-3 days. Others present with symptoms of the nervous system.

In the non-paralytic form, the person is irritable and has fever, headache, vomiting, and generalized pain and stiffness. This may last for a week or two and the person is normal again. In the paralytic form, in addition to the symptoms of nonparalytic form, the person has weakness of various groups of muscles, with the loss of reflexes. The individual may be hypersensitive to touch. Loss of bladder control and constipation may be present. If the cranial nerves are affected, the facial muscles may be weak. There may be difficulty in swallowing. Polio affecting the brainstem region may result in difficulty in breathing. There is no loss of sensation or mental function.

Following the acute infectious stage, there may be improvement due to the recovery of undamaged neurons that had been compressed by the edema produced by inflammation. Neurons that are damaged result in chronic signs of muscle atrophy and paralysis. The loss of function of muscles can slow down the growth of bone in children producing shortening of a limb. Disuse of the joint and soft tissue in the affected limb can lead to joint stiffness and contractures of the soft tissue.

Risk factors:

The chances of paralysis after infection is increased during pregnancy, old age, excessive physical exertion, tonsillectomy or tooth extraction, or vaccination - all factors that tend to lower the immunity or ease the entry of the virus into the blood and lymph.

Caution and Recommendations to Therapists:

Polio can be spread by "carriers" or during the incubation period and early signs of infection. Massage should be avoided at all costs during the acute stages of the disease.

Massage therapists are more likely to encounter adults in the chronic non infective stage of the disease. The aim is to retain joint mobility and prevent contractures. Position the affected area of the client in a neutral position. You may need to support the area with pillows. The paralysis of one group of muscles results in overactivity of the antagonist muscle and increased tone. The increased tone in turn, results in excessive stretch and scarring of the affected group. Passively move joints through the full range of motion. Use transverse friction movements over joints and atrophied muscle. Strokes like effleurage and petrissage can increase the circulation in these unused areas. Remember that the loss of motor function is permanent.

The loss of nerve supply to the area may be associated with dryness and fragility of skin. Do not use vigorous massage or excessive pressure. Edema may be present in the affected limb. Keep the limb elevated and use lymphatic drainage techniques. Concentrate massage strokes on muscles that are stressed by the alteration of posture to compensate for the paralyzed muscle groups. Look for pressure ulcers and skin changes in people who wear braces or use crutches. Avoid massaging these areas. Refer client to local support groups (see Appendix IV).

Notes: ─────────────────────────────────────

Polio vaccines are given as oral drops and is 90 % effective in preventing the disease. However, the vaccine should be avoided in people with lowered immunity.

Posterior compartment syndrome

Musculoskeletal system

A collection of signs and symptoms produced by increased pressure and consequent reduced blood flow to a closed muscle compartment in the leg.

Cause:

In the calf ie. in the region posterior to the tibia and the fibula, the muscles are compartmentalized into two by a thick fascia (connective tissue sheath). This sheath separates the gastrocnemius and soleus muscles into a superficial compartment, and the tibialis posterior, flexor hallucis longus and flexor digitorum longus into a deeper compartment.

Any condition that increases the pressure in either of these compartments compromises in the blood flow to the soft tissue. The ischemia, inflammation and swelling in the compartment produce the characteristic symptoms.

Signs and Symptoms:

There is a gradual onset of pain in the calf. The pain increases on using the limb and comes on after the same amount of exertion every time. Often, both legs are affected.

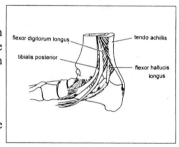

Risk factors:

Overuse, and repetitive use of the muscles in the compartment result in this condition.

Caution and Recommendations to Massage Therapists:

The limb should be placed in level with the heart. Elevation may reduce the blood flow to the already compromised tissue. Placing the limb in a dependent position may increase the venous congestion due to the effect of gravity. In the acute stage, measures to reduce the inflammation and swelling are helpful. Rest and ice application have been found to be beneficial. The thighs should be massaged well, using broad strokes like effleurage and petrissage to increase venous and lymphatic drainage.

In the subacute stage, heat can be applied to soften the connective tissue. Suitable strokes such as cross fibre friction are used to stretch the tight fascia. However, such techniques should be avoided if it is too painful. In those with lowered sensation, care should be taken not to use excessive pressure as the feedback from the client is likely to be inadequate.

Notes:

The condition is diagnosed by measuring the pressure in the compartment. If the symptoms are chronic or severe, surgery may be done to reduce the pressure.

Portal Hypertension

Gastrointestinal system

An abnormal increase of pressure in the portal circulation. The portal circulation is responsible for carrying blood from the abdominal organs into the liver before it flows into the inferior vena cava and the right side of the heart.

Cause:

Any condition that blocks or obstructs the flow of blood in the portal or hepatic veins can cause this. The portal vein can be occluded by structures around it like enlarged lymph nodes or tumors. Thrombosis in the vein can also cause obstruction. The most common cause of portal hypertension is cirrhosis of the liver where the fibrous bands formed in cirrhosis distort the hepatic blood vessels. In severe right heart failure, there is damming of blood in the veins leading to this condition.

Signs and Symptoms:

The signs and symptoms are produced by the damming of blood in the veins in the abdomen. The increase in pressure forces fluid from the abdominal capillaries into the peritoneal cavity (ascites). It also results in the blood seeking alternate routes to reach the heart. Dilatation of collateral vessels in the lower end of the esophagus, around the umbilicus and rectum occurs. Rupture and bleeding of these dilated and tortuous vessels can be fatal (see Esophageal varices). Portal hypertension also causes the spleen to enlarge.

Risk factors:

Risk factors of thrombus formation, chronic alcohol intake and any condition that causes cirrhosis predisposes an individual to portal hypertension.

Caution and Recommendations to Therapists:

A gentle, soothing massage avoiding the abdomen is recommended. Do not try to reduce the edema present in the lower limbs in these individuals. Usually, Portal hypertension is associated with cirrhosis of the liver and liver failure. Jaundice, anemia, easy bruisability and susceptibility to infection are all associated.

Notes:

The primary concern is to avoid bleeding from the dilated collateral veins. Sclerosing agents are used to occlude the veins in the esophagus which are prone to hemorrhage extensively. Surgery to shunt the blood from the portal vein, bypassing the obstruction is also resorted to.

Premenstrual syndrome (PMS)

Reproductive system

The physical and psychological symptoms perceived 3-14 days prior to the onset of menstruation.

Cause:

The cause has been attributed to a complex interaction between various factors. Excess levels of estrogen, prolactin, changes in estrogen-progesterone ratio, stress, hypoglycemia are some of the factors. Increased levels of aldosterone, decreased levels of dopamine and serotonin, deficiency of vitamin B12 have also been implicated.

Signs and Symptoms:

The breasts are painful and swollen. Headache, backache, changes in co-ordination, abdominal pain and a bloated feeling are other symptoms. The person may have craving for sweets. Psychologically, the individual may become depressed, irritable, and anxious with inability to concentrate. Other behavioral changes may also be seen. The symptoms and signs are different from woman to woman and from cycle to cycle in the same person.

Risk factors:

It is more common in women above the age of 30.

Caution and Recommendations to Therapists:

Since the exact cause of PMS is not known a variety of treatments are available, of which relaxation techniques is one. A relaxing and gentle whole body massage is indicated. Use of essential oils like lavender, chamomile, rose in a 5% dilution are recommended by some. Warm compresses to the back and lower abdomen helps reduce pain and tenderness. Some therapists advocate breast massage. This should be done only after obtaining an informed consent from the client and only if the therapist is comfortable and has had training in this area. Cold towel breast wrap which reduce congestion by vasoconstriction of the blood vessels are also used. Lymphatic drainage techniques with strokes directed towards the axillary lymph nodes are additional techniques used to reduce congestion and breast tenderness. Rhythmic, slow strokes using broad surface techniques like palmar kneading are used to massage the pectoralis major and minor muscles underlying the breast.

Notes: ──

PMS is treated symptomatically with pain killers, regular exercise and dietary changes. Diets low in simple sugars, high in lean meat, avoidance of caffeine are some dietary measures used. In severe cases, hormones are given.

Prostatitis

Reproductive system

An inflammation of the prostate.

Cause:

It is usually caused by bacteria. However, the inflammation may occur after catheterization or using an instrument in the area.

Signs and Symptoms:

High fever with chills, muscle and joint pain are common. There is frequency and urgency on passing urine. The urine may be cloudy. A dull ache may be present in the low back and perineal area.

Risk factors:

Catheterisation, use of instruments in the area are all predisposing factors. It is more common in males with diabetes mellitus.

Caution and Recommendations to Therapists:

The prostate is more deeply placed and cannot be approached from the surface of the body. A light, soothing full body massage helps. Encourage client to take the full course of antibiotics prescribed.

Notes: ────────────────────────────────

Prostatic Hyperplasia

A benign enlargement of the prostate.

Cause:

It is caused by changes in the level of hormones as a person ages.

Signs and Symptoms:

The symptoms are due to the narrowing of the urethra as the middle lobe of the prostate enlarges and compresses the urethra. The person has urgency and difficulty in passing urine.

Risk factors:

It is common with aging.

Caution and Recommendations to Therapists:

The prostate cannot be accessed from the exterior of the body. A full body massage is given for general relaxation. Encourage client to seek medical help.

Notes: ────────────────────────────────

This condition causes stagnation of urine making the urinary bladder, urethra and kidneys more susceptible to infection. Benign prostatic hyperplasia is treated with surgery. Sometimes drugs are given to block the action of the sympathetics. The side effect of this is postural hypotension.

Psoriasis

A chronic, relapsing, inflammatory disease of the skin.

Cause:

The cause is unknown. The rate at which the keratinocytes (from the basal layer of the skin) migrate to the superficial layer is faster than normal in these individuals.

Signs and Symptoms:

The clients present with patches of different sizes with whitish or yellowish scales which are loosely adherent to the epidermis of the skin. There is redness around these patches. The patches give the appearance of drops of mortar on the skin. The patches may persist throughout life with periods of remission and exacerbation. There are many forms of Psoriasis. In the more common form - psoriasis vulgaris, the patches are typically seen in the elbow, knee and scalp. In eruptive psoriasis the patches are smaller and seen in the trunk and limbs. In pustular psoriasis, the lesions have pustules and there is generalized fever. These patches occur even in the soles of feet and the palms. Oval or annular psoriasis is a rare form.

Risk factors:

It commonly occurs in adults above 30 years of age. There is also a genetic predisposition. In individuals who are predisposed, skin trauma or alcohol consumption, may precipitate an attack.

Caution and Recommendations to Therapists:

Psoriaisis, although unsightly, is not contagious and massage can be beneficial. The scales which are loosely adherent may dislodge with massage and be a nuisance to the therapist. Since there is no known cure for psoriasis the clients may be on varied treatment regimens. Some clients may be on topical corticosteroid treatment which makes the local area susceptible to superinfection by bacteria. Take care to wash hands thoroughly before massaging such individuals. Other treatment regimens used such as methotrexate or cyclosporine suppress the general immunity of the individuals and make them susceptible to infection. Do not massage such clients when you harbor a cold, cough or any other mild form of infection. Schedule their appointment at a time when they are unlikely to come in contact with other clients who may have an infection. Refer clients to local support groups (see Appendix IV for resources).

Notes:

Pulmonary embolism

A blockage of a pulmonary artery by thrombus or a foreign substance.

Cause:

It is commonly caused by a thrombus that has been dislodged from a leg vein. However, thrombus can be from other veins too. Rarely, the thrombus can be fat, air or tumor cells. Prolonged blockage can lead to death of lung tissue (pulmonary infarction).

Signs and Symptoms:

Large emboli that occlude the artery totally can be fatal. Smaller emboli produce difficulty in breathing, cough with blood tinged sputum and chest pain. Low grade fever may be present. Depending on the size of the emboli, the symptoms vary. Blue coloration of fingers and toes may be seen indicating reduced oxygenation of blood. The neck veins may appear prominent.

Risk factors:

Conditions which tend to reduce flow of blood as in prolonged immobilization, heart failure, varicose veins, thrombophlebitis (infection/inflammation of veins) and obesity can predispose to embolism. Increased clotting tendencies of blood as during pregnancy, oral contraceptives and after severe burns also make a person prone for emboli. Fat emboli can be a complication of surgery and fractures. Conditions that thicken the blood (polycythemia) such as severe burns, can also speed up emboli formation. Emboli are more common in the older age group.

Caution and Recommendations to Therapists:

Do not massage vigorously, the legs of individuals with moderate to severe varicose veins, or those who have been immobilized for a long time, or those pregnant. Vigorous massage in individuals who are predisposed may result in dislodgment of thrombi already formed.

Those clients with a previous history of emboli are likely to be on anti-coagulant therapy and are prone to bleed easily. Do not use excess pressure while massaging these individuals. Early mobilization after surgery helps avoid thrombi and emboli formation. Encourage clients in plaster casts or those advised prolonged bed rest to passively or actively move joints that are not immobilized.

Notes:

Small emboli are treated with oxygen and drugs to reduce coagulation (clotting) of blood.

Raynaud's syndrome

Intense spasm of arteries and arterioles in the fingers or toes.

Cause:

The cause of Primary Raynaud's syndrome is unknown, and may be precipitated by cold, strong emotions or stress. It is thought to be due to hyperactivity of the sympathetic nervous system. Secondary Raynaud's phenomenon can be associated with frost bite, occupations using heavy vibrating equipment or requiring frequent exposure of limbs to alternating temperatures of cold and warmth (eg. butchers, caterers), collagen disorders (eg. Systemic Lupus Erythematosus), neurological disorders and disorders which tend to occlude arteries.

Signs and Symptoms:

The client may present with slight swelling of fingers or toes. The reduced blood flow to these parts result in change of skin color — pale or cyanosed (blue). The client may complain of loss of sensations, or tingling. Following the ischemia (reduced blood flow) the part may become pink (hyperemia). The nails may appear brittle and the skin of the fingers or toes may be thickened. In late stages, ulcers or gangrene may be seen (see Appendix I figure 4 and 15).

Risk factors:

Those in occupations using vibrating equipment or those requiring frequent exposure to alternating cold and heat are at higher risk. Smoking has been shown to be associated with this disease.

Caution and Recommendations to Therapists:

Recurrent washing of hands with alternating cold and warm water should be avoided. Massage helps clients with Raynaud's by increasing blood flow to the periphery. By reducing stress, massage helps lower sympathetic stimulation and thereby relax the smooth muscles of blood vessels. Do not apply heat packs to affected areas during an attack of spasm.

Notes:

Renal failure

A condition where the kidney is unable to fulfill its' function according to the demands made by the body.

Cause:

Renal failure could be acute (sudden onset) or chronic (occurs over a number of years). There are many causes of acute renal failure. The causes may be classified as those due to conditions other than the urinary tract - *prerenal*; those due to kidney disease - *renal*; and those due to problems with the drainage of urine from the kidney - *postrenal*.

Prerenal conditions affect the renal function by altering the blood flow to the kidney. Intrarenal conditions damage the kidney tissue. Postrenal causes are conditions that obstruct the outflow of urine and produce damage to the kidney by backpressure.

Normal Urine	
Volume	1.5 liters/day (approx.)
Glucose	0
Albumin	0 - trace
Urea	25 - 35/24 hrs.
Specific gravity	1.003 - 1.03
pH	5 - 8
Bacteria	< 100,000 organisms/ml.

Chronic renal failure is caused by conditions that destroy the nephrons - the functional unit of the kidney. It may be a complication of untreated acute renal failure. Systemic diseases like diabetes mellitus, prolonged hypertension and hereditary defects of the kidney can lead to this.

Signs and Symptoms:

Acute renal failure is usually reversible and can be treated effectively if diagnosed early. There is a sudden decrease in urine formation. The retention of fluid causes edema. The accumulation of urea, and other toxic substances, alteration in sodium, calcium and potassium levels have their own detrimental effects on the body.

Renal failure has effects on practically all systems. There is nausea, vomiting, diarrhea or constipation, bleeding from the gut (gastrointestinal system). Accumulation of fluid can cause pulmonary edema and difficulty in breathing (respiratory system). There is anemia, hypotension and finally heart failure (cardiovascular system). The skin is dry and pale, with a tendency to bruise easily. Itching is also present (integumentary system). The person is irritable and confused (nervous system). The bones are osteoporotic and prone to fracture easily (musculoskeletal system). Impotence, alterations in menstrual cycle and other sexual dysfunctions are common (reproductive system).

Risk factors:

Prerenal: Dehydration (diarrhea, vomiting, burns), loss of large quantities of blood, or heart failure can predispose to this type.

Renal: Exposure to drugs and chemicals that are toxic to the kidney eg. antibiotics like gentamycin, kanamycin and heavy metals like lead and mercury and autoimmune reactions like glomerulonephritis increase the risk.

Postrenal: Obstruction to the ureter by renal stones, prostatic hyperplasia and narrowing of the urethra can result in this type of failure.

Caution and Recommendations to Therapists:

Obtain a detailed history as to the cause of the renal failure and alter treatment accordingly.

A light, soothing full body massage of short duration is recommended. The edema produced is a compensatory mechanism for the excess fluid that have been retained in the body. Therefore the massage should not be directed to reduce the edema. This may overload the heart that is already stressed by the fluid retention. The oil used helps reduce the dryness and itching of the skin. Only light pressure should be used as these individuals bruise easily. Also, the bones are fragile and may fracture even with moderate pressure.

If the person is on dialysis, avoid massage over a wide area around the infusion site.

Individuals who have had renal transplants may be on drugs that suppress immunity. Avoid massage if harboring even a mild form of infection.

Notes: _____

The major functions of the kidney are to remove the end products of metabolism from the blood and to regulate the levels of fluid, electrolytes and thereby the pH of the body fluids. Other functions include secretion of hormones that regulate the formation of red blood cells (erythropoietin) and blood pressure (renin). It also plays a major role in the conversion of Vitamin D to an active form. Vitamin D participates in the regulation of calcium and phosphates.

Renal stones (Kidney stones, Renal calculi, Nephrolithiasis)

Renal system

Formation of solitary or multiple stones in the pelvis of the kidney.

Cause:

Stones are formed in the kidney when the urine is saturated with material that it normally excretes eg. calcium salts, uric acid, cystine, magnesium ammonium phosphate. This material tends to precipitate in the absence of substances that normally inhibit precipitation. A substance called nephrocalcin that has been recently identified is a natural inhibitor of precipitation. Precipitation is also promoted if organic material from the epithelium lining the tubules act as a nucleus or nidus for stone formation.

Signs and Symptoms:

Pain is the most common symptom. Excruciating, colicky pain in the upper outer quadrant of the abdomen and the flanks are common. The pain may be referred to the lower abdomen, scrotum/labia and inner thigh (see Appendicitis for locations of referred pain). It may be intense enough to cause nausea and vomiting. The skin may be cold and clammy. Small particles may be seen in the urine if the stone is excreted. The urine may be pink due to the presence of blood (hematuria).

Risk factors:

Excessive bone resorption caused by immobility, bone disease and hyperparathyroidism predispose to calcium stones. Gout promotes formation of uric acid stones. Alkaline urine promotes formation of magnesium ammonium phosphate stones. A common cause of alkaline urine is bacterial infection. Any condition that predisposes to stagnation of urine also promotes stone formation.

Caution and Recommendations to Therapists:

Encourage the client to alter diet according to the type of stone identified by physician and increase the intake of fluid. Massage is beneficial in reducing the pain and stress.

Notes:

Dietary alterations can be made to prevent the recurrence of stone formation. To prevent calcium oxalate stones, diets rich in oxalate such as spinach, cocoa, chocolate, pecans, peanuts may be avoided. To prevent uric acid stones, high purine containing foods such as anchovies, liver, sardines, kidneys, sweetbreads, lentils and alcohol (especially beer and wine) should be avoided.

Urinary stones that are smaller than 5mm are excreted in the urine spontaneously. Larger stones may have to be removed surgically. Extracorporeal shock wave lithotripsy - a procedure that uses shock waves to breakup the stones into tiny pieces small enough to be excreted in the urine is a popular form of treatment. Prevention of recurrence, however, should be the major goal.

Respiratory Distress Syndrome (RDS, Hyaline Membrane Disease)

Respiratory system

A condition in infants, that produces difficulty in breathing due to the lack of a lipoprotein -surfactant, in the lungs.

Cause:

The normal lung produces a lipoprotein called surfactant that reduces the surface tension in the lung and allows the lung to expand easily on inspiration. In this condition, surfactant is lacking. This results in difficulty in inflating the lung and collapse of segments of lung (atelectasis).

Signs and Symptoms:

There is difficulty in breathing. The respiratory rate is rapid and labored and grunting may be present. If severe, the heart rate is rapid and cyanosis (blue coloration of the mucous membrane) may be seen.

Risk factors:

Premature infants, infants born to diabetic mothers, infants delivered by Cesarean section are at risk.

Caution and Recommendations to Therapists:

Infants who have had this problem may take up to a year to recover - depending on the severity. Consult Pediatrician before massage.

Notes: _____

Rheumatic Heart disease (Rheumatic fever)

Cardiovascular, Musculoskeletal systems

An inflammatory disease affecting many systems following a streptococcal bacterial infection.

Cause:

It is due to the reaction of antibodies produced against the specific bacteria (viz. group A beta hemolytic streptococci), attacking other body tissues. The heart and the joints are most commonly affected.

Signs and Symptoms:

Typically, the person gives a history of sore throat a few days to 6 week before the onset of symptoms. There is fever and joint pain that seems to migrate from one large joint to another. Signs of inflammation - redness, swelling, loss of function, and warmth are seen in the affected joint. A rash may accompany these symptoms. Firm nodules (rounded masses) may be present under the skin. If the nervous system is affected, there may be symptoms of hyperirritability, inability to concentrate, abnormal writhing movements of the limb, among others. Often there is inflammation of the valves of the heart, which on resolving by fibrosis, causes narrowing or leakiness of valves.

Risk factors:

The incidence is higher in the lower socioeconomic group. It is more common in children between the ages of 5-15. Higher incidence is seen in the winter and early spring.

Caution and Recommendations to Therapists:

A detailed history should be taken in order to ascertain the extent of the disease. In acute cases, measures to decrease pain and swelling in the joints may be taken. In chronic cases, treatment should be modified according to the extent of the disease.

Notes: _____

In the acute stage, it is treated with antibiotics and strict bed rest.

Ringworm (Tinea, Dermatophytoses)

Integumentary system

A fungal infection of the skin.

Cause:

A type of fungus - mold which have long, hollow, branching filaments, causes this disease. The fungus thrives on the cooler surface of the skin. Different fungi affect different areas. Fungal infection of the body is called tinea corporis, scalp-tinea capitis, hands-tinea manus, feet-tinea pedis (athlete's foot), nails-tinea unguium, groin and upper thighs-tinea cruris or jock itch.

Signs and Symptoms:

Tinea corporis appears as round or oval patches with a central clear area surrounded by a red border with pustules. Itching is pronounced. Many such lesions can be found all over the body. (see Appendix 1 figure 13)

Tinea capitis appears as painless, round, hairless patches on the scalp. Itching may be present. The lesion may appear red, with scaling.

Tinea pedis (athlete's foot) affect the spaces between the toes and appear as scaly lesions, or inflamed, oozing, painful lesions. Foul smells and itching may also be present.

In tinea unguium the nails become opaque or silvery, yellow or brown. The nails soon thicken and crack. In tinea manus, a blister appears in the palm of the hand or on the finger. Chronic lesions may appear dry and scaly.

Risk factors:

Fungal infections are common in people with lowered immunity. Tinea pedis is more common in clients whose feet are constantly damp due to sweating or who wear occlusive shoes. Children are more prone to tinea capitis. Tinea corporis affects people of all ages and is transmitted from pet animals and other affected individuals.

Caution and Recommendations for Therapists:

Massage is contraindicated as the infection spreads by contact. Boil and steam press clothes, towels and bedding if contact has been made.

Notes: _____

Fungal infections can be treated, but require prolonged treatment sometimes lasting for six to twelve months.

Salpingitis

Reproductive system

An inflammation of the fallopian tubes.

Cause:

It is commonly caused by the organism Chlamydia trachomatis or N. Gonorrheoeae which are sexually transmitted. The infection reaches the fallopian tube via the vagina, cervix and endometrium.

Signs and Symptoms:

The person has lower abdominal pain, pain on passing urine, fever and white discharge from the vagina. The lower abdomen feels tender and rigid. There may be pain on having intercourse. The tube heals by fibrosis causing adhesions between organs in the pelvis and/or blockage of the tube - a common cause of infertility.

Risk factors:

It is more common in sexually active women between the ages of 15-20. It is also common in those who use intrauterine devices for contraception or who have abnormal development of the reproductive organs. Oro-genital contact, vaginal or rectal intercourse with an infected person increases the risk of contracting the disease.

Caution and Recommendations to Therapists:

Encourage the client to take the full course of the prescribed antibiotics. Educate the client that sexual partners may also have to be treated to prevent reinfection. Avoid abdominal area while massaging the client. The client may feel more comfortable in a position with the head and knee raised with pillows. There is no scope for transmission of infection as it is sexually transmitted. Ask the client to keep underclothes on during massage. The standard precautions for any infection should be taken (see Appendix II).

Notes:

It is treated with high doses of antibiotics for 14 days. Babies born to infected mothers may be infected and the organism can cause conjunctivitis in the babies.

Scabies
Integumentary system

An itchy skin infection produced by mites.

Cause:

Scabies is a disease that is caused by a mite - Sarcoptes scabei. The mite burrows into the epidermis and these burrows along with the fecal matter of the mite are responsible for the itching. The females lay eggs in the burrows which hatch in 3-5 days thus restarting the cycle again.

Signs and symptoms:

The client presents with severe itching especially between the fingers, flexor surface of the wrist, axilla, gluteal creases, thigh, genital areas and other areas of the body. There may be secondary bacterial infection as a result of injury produced by scratching. Small reddish vesicles can be seen in these areas.

Risk factors:

It affects people of all socioeconomic groups.

Caution and Recommendations to Therapists:

Massage is contraindicated because scabies is contagious. However scabies is treatable.

It is possible to contract scabies by sharing clothes, bedding or towels of an infected person. Do not massage a client even with a suspicion of scabies. If you have come in contact, apply the prescribed Lindane lotion or cream (Kwell) all over the body and wash after 12 hours. Repeat treatment if necessary. Wash all linen and clothes in boiling hot soapy water and detergent.

Since scabies is very contagious, it is advisable to cancel all appointments for the day if you have treated an infected client inadvertently. Although the mite can survive outside the body for only a few hours, disinfect the furniture and all linen likely to have come in contact with the client with scabies.

Notes: _____

Sciatic nerve lesions

Nervous system

A condition resulting from pressure or injury to the sciatic nerve.

Cause:

This is most commonly caused by prolapse of the disc (herniated disc, slipped disc) with pressure on the nerve roots (L4, L5, S1, S2, S3) that give rise to the nerve. It may also be caused by narrowing of the intervertebral canal due to hypertrophy of the facets of the vertebrae. Congenital abnormality of the vertebrae can also produce this. Trauma, gunshot wounds, fracture vertebrae are other causes. The sciatic nerve can also be injured or compressed after it's exit from the spinal cord as in spasm of the piriformis muscle which lies over the nerve. Improper administration of injections in the gluteal region can injure the sciatic nerve. The nerve can also be injured anywhere along its long course as it travels from the gluteal region, behind the thigh, behind the knee in the popliteal fossa and as it divides into the common peroneal nerve that goes around the neck of the fibula to the anterior compartment, and the tibial nerve which descends in the calf region to the plantar aspect of the foot.

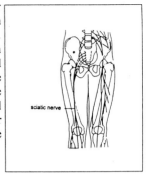

sciatic nerve

Signs and Symptoms:

The signs and symptoms vary according to the location of the lesion. If the sciatic nerve is injured close to the spinal cord then the person has difficulty in voluntarily flexing the knee (supply to the hamstrings affected), dorsiflexion and plantar flexion of the ankle (loss of nerve supply to the tibialis anterior, peroneal muscles, gastrocnemius and soleus). Movement of toes are also affected (nerve supply to the extensor and flexor muscles of the toes lost). The extension and abduction of the hip is weak.

The muscles supplied by the nerve are atrophic and have decreased tone. The person tends to swing the foot up and bring it with a slap onto the ground due to the tendency of the foot to drop (footdrop). The sensations to the lateral aspect of the leg below the level of the knee as well as to the foot is reduced. Deep sensations such as joint and position sense is also lost. The autonomic function is also affected resulting in reduced circulation to the region. Sweating and temperature regulation is poor in this region.

If the injury is lower, flexion of the knee is present. But movement and sensations of the ankle are affected. If only the common peroneal is injured, dorsiflexion of the foot is impaired with loss of sensation in the anterior and lateral aspect of the leg and between the toes on the dorsum of the foot. Injury only to the tibial nerve results in impaired plantar flexion of the foot with difficulty in abducting and adducting the toes. The sensations are affected on the plantar surface as well as the lateral aspect of the foot.

Risk factors:

See Cause.

Caution and Recommendations to Therapists:

Assess the motor and sensory function and keep a record of it. The extent of the loss can be kept on record using diagrams of outline of the legs and coloring areas where sensory and motor loss is present. An idea of the cause of the lesion can be obtained by a good history. Treatment should be modified according to the cause (eg. disc prolapse, piriformis spasm). For the muscles involved, the aim is to increase tone, reduce atrophy, prevent contractures and reduce edema. Pressure ulcers have to be watched for and prevented. Joint stiffness should be prevented or reduced.

Position the limb neutrally and elevate it above the level of the heart to use the effect of gravity to reduce edema. The foot should be supported with pillows to maintain a neutral position ie. not excessively dorsiflexed or plantar flexed. The client can be positioned half prone or lying on the side as the affected area is on the posterior and lateral aspect of the leg. Since the sensation is reduced, excessive pressure and force should not be used. Passively move all joints (do not forget the small joints of the toes) through as wide a range of motion as possible without using force. Use transverse friction around joints. A stimulatory massage helps to increase the tone of the muscles. Use broad strokes of effleurage and petrissage to increase circulation and lymph drainage. Lymph drainage techniques can be used to reduce edema. Massage the stressed muscles of the pelvis, back and neck which are overused to compensate for the lack of muscle control over the leg. Avoid massaging a wide area around pressure ulcers if present. Work in close conjunction with a physiotherapist.

Notes: _____

Scleroderma (Dermatosclerosis, Sclerema, Scleroma, Scleriasis, Hide Bound Disease, Systemic sclerosis)

Integumentary system

A progressive, widespread disease of the connective tissue.

Cause:

The cause is not known. It may be due to the immunity of the body attacking tissues of self (autoimmune disease).

Signs and Symptoms:

This disease typically begins with vascular changes such as pallor, blue coloration or redness of the skin. Slowly, there is thickening of the skin through fibrosis. This fibrosis may fix the skin to the deeper tissues like the fascia covering tendons and muscle. The lesion may develop rapidly or as is more common gradually in a single or multiple area. It may be well localized or diffuse and ill defined, level, depressed or slightly elevated from the normal skin. The skin feels thick and leathery and cannot be pinched up in folds. The surface of the skin is usually smooth, but may be slightly scaly or nodular. The shrinking and progressive thickening of the skin may greatly interfere with the function and nutrition of the parts beneath producing pain, edema and calcification. The muscles may atrophy as a result and the joints stiffen.

If the thickening is over the hands and fingers (sclerodactylia) the hands become stiff, immobile and useless. If over the chest, respiration may be compromised. If on the face, the natural folds disappear. Movements of the mouth and eyelids are inhibited and the person has a mask like face. In some cases, the infiltration disappears gradually leaving a dry, wrinkled and parchment-like skin. This condition is systemic and can involve the central nervous system, lungs, esophagus, heart, duodenum and kidneys (see Appendix 1 figure 11).

Risk factors:

It is more common in women, African-Americans, in youth and the middle aged.

Caution and Recommendations to Therapists:

It is not contagious. Local massage with oil or a mildly stimulating ointment is very beneficial. Friction strokes can reduce adhesions. Deeper strokes help increase circulation to the local area and improve nutrition and drainage. Passive and active movements of the joints help retain the range of movement. The individual may be on corticosteroids or immunosuppressants which lower the immunity. Ensure that they are not exposed to even mild forms of infection in the clinic as such infections can have serious consequences in these immuno-compromised individuals. Refer client to local groups (see Appendix).

Notes: ─────────────────────────────────────

There is no cure for this condition. Immunosuppressants and corticosteroids are used to reduce symptoms.

Scoliosis Musculoskeletal system

Bending of the vertebral column to one side with or without rotation of the bodies of the vertebrae.

Cause:

There is no known cause in general, but in some it may follow diseases like poliomyelitis, congenitally deformed vertebra, neurofibromatosis and cerebral palsy. Scoliosis may be compensatory to other deformities such as those of neck, arms, legs of uneven length, unilateral paralysis of muscles, injury to the spine and unilateral lung disease.

Signs and Symptoms:

It is noted by the deformity such as a high shoulder, prominent hip or protruding scapula. Pain may be caused by the pressure on the ribs or the pelvis. The crowding of the intraabdominal structures may produce symptoms. There may be difficulty in breathing when the movement of the ribs is impaired by the deformity. Low back pain may be present due to the compensation made by muscles to maintain the posture. Of the two types of scoliosis, the postural type is a small curvature that corrects with bending. The structural type is one where the deformity is fixed.

Risk factors:

Scoliosis is more frequent in adolescence and is more common in girls. In some there is a family history of scoliosis. Habitual asymmetric posture related to certain occupations can result in this condition.

Caution and Recommendations to Therapists:

Work in conjunction with the physician and physiotherapist. A thorough assessment is necessary to identify the extent of scoliosis, associated trigger points and spasm of muscles. The role of the massage therapist is to relax tense muscles, and increase blood flow to the fatigued muscles. The client should be positioned

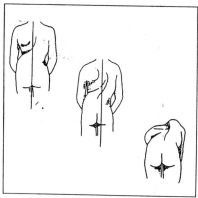

according to individual comfort and supported with pillows wherever necessary. In the postural type, the aim is to restore muscle tone and relax tense muscles while correcting the posture. Massage groups of muscles in the legs, lower back and gluteals that are put under excessive strain while the client maintains balance. Heat packs help alleviate low back pain. Deep muscle stripping, fascial work and joint mobilizations are other forms of therapy that should be used to stretch the shortened structures. Deep diaphragmatic breathing should also be employed to improve thoracic mobility.

Encourage client to do remedial exercises to maintain range of motion and to correct muscle imbalances. The frequency of massage should be varied according to the type of scoliosis. Initially, more frequent massages should be scheduled for postural/functional type of scoliosis, with the frequency reduced as the individual improves. For the structural type, massages are given once a week over a very long period.

Physiotherapy is a major component of treating structural curves. Severe cases of structural scoliosis may require corrective surgery and/or braces. Refer client to local support groups (see Appendix IV).

Notes: _____

Scoliosis is classified as functional, postural, nonstructural or first degree scoliosis if it is due to muscular imbalance. This type can be corrected with exercises. Structural, second or third degree scoliosis refers to scoliosis caused by bony or connective tissue changes. This type is harder to correct.

Seasonal Affective Disorder (SAD)

Nervous system

A periodic major depression which manifests at specific seasons.

Cause:

It is thought to be due to a dysfunction of the natural biological rhythm. It has been associated with changes in hormonal secretions and certain neurotransmitters in the brain. Changes in sleep patterns have also been observed in people with depression.

Signs and Symptoms:

Episodes of depression occur in these individuals during the winter time when the days are short and periods of darkness are longer. There is a marked reduction in the depression when the duration of light in the day becomes longer. The person exhibits easy fatiguability, loss of interest in every day and pleasurable activities and insomnia. In severe depression, suicide may be attempted.

Risk factors:

It is common in people living in the northern latitudes. There may be a family history of depression.

Caution and Recommendations to Therapists:

A general relaxation massage is recommended. Encourage the client to take the prescribed medications.

Notes: _____

It is treated with exposure to intense white light at a specified time of day for a specific duration. Antidepressants are also used.

Shin splints (Idiopathic compartment syndrome)

Inflammation of the proximal portion of any of the musculotendinous units originating from the lower part of the tibia.

Cause:

Repetitive stress of the muscles arising from the lower tibia may produce this condition. It may involve the group of muscles anterolateral to the tibia (tibialis anterior, extensor hallucis longus, extensor digitorum longus) or those posteromedial to it.

Signs and Symptoms:

The person complains of pain and tenderness lateral to the tibia if the anterolateral muscles are involved. The pain is increased on dorsiflexing the foot. The pain is localized to the posteromedial aspects of the lower tibial region, in the posteromedial type. In the later, the pain is increased on standing on the toes. There may be signs of inflammation viz. redness, swelling and warmth. The muscles surrounding the area may be in spasm with increased tone and trigger points. Weakness of the involved muscles may be seen in chronic cases. A common complication of shin splint is stress fractures.

Risk factors:

Using shoes with hard heels, recurrent contact of heel on a hard surface as in running on hard, uneven or inclined surfaces, overzealous training, can predispose to anterolateral shinsplint. Ballet or other sports involving plantar flexion predispose to the posteromedial type.

Caution and Recommendations to Therapists:

In acute cases, the limb should be rested for 2-3 days. Apply icepacks, and elevate limb to reduce swelling and inflammation. Later, use friction massage to increase blood flow and prevent adhesions. Gentle stretching also helps. Refer to physiotherapist for strengthening exercises.

Initially, short treatments lasting for half an hour are recommended at a frequency of two to three times per week.

Notes:

Shock

Profound and widespread reduction in the delivery of oxygen and nutrients to tissues.

Cause:

It is caused by any condition that affects the volume of blood pumped out of the heart per minute (cardiac output), and/or the resistance offered by the blood vessels to the flow of blood. Shock can be classified according to the cause as cardiogenic shock (due to abnormalities in the heart), extracardiac obstructive shock (conditions like fluid in the pericardium, pulmonary embolism, that affect outflow), oligemic shock (reduced blood volume as in hemorrhage, dehydration), distributive shock (conditions like infection in the blood, overdose of toxic products, severe allergic reaction - anaphylactic shock, sympathetic nervous system inactivity, endocrine disorders etc.).

Signs and Symptoms:

It is characterized by a lowered blood pressure, disorientation, palpitation, cold and clammy skin. Depending on the type of shock other symptoms may be present.

Risk factors:

See Cause.

Caution and Recommendations to Therapists:

Shock is an emergency as it can produce irreversible damage to the brain if continued for sometime. If you suspect shock in a client in your clinic call for medical help immediately. Loosen the clothes and allow client to be in a recumbent position with the leg end elevated until help arrives.

Notes: ──

Sinusitis

An inflammation of the paranasal sinuses.

Cause:

It is usually caused by a viral or bacterial infection. Sinusitis may also be a complication of common cold or allergy. The congestion of the nose results in blockage of the opening of the sinus into the nasal cavity and a build up of pressure in the sinus. There is a slow absorption of the air in the sinus and a partial vacuum is formed. All these processes are responsible for the characteristic symptoms.

Signs and Symptoms:

The symptoms are similar in acute and chronic sinusitis. There is nasal congestion followed by a mucous or purulent discharge from the nose. There is pain localized to specific areas depending on the sinus affected. If the maxillary sinus is affected there is pain over the cheeks and upper teeth. If ethmoid, over the eyes, if frontal, over the eyebrow and if sphenoid, the pain is felt behind the eye.

frontal sinus

maxillary sinus

Risk factors:

Any condition which interferes with the drainage and movement of air in the sinuses can predispose to sinusitis. It is more common in individuals with deviated nasal septum, nasal polyps, diabetes, nasal intubation, immunosuppressed individuals and those using steroids over prolonged periods. Swimming in contaminated water also predisposes to this condition.

Caution and Recommendations to Therapists:

Local application of heat helps relieve pain. Encourage clients to complete the full course of antibiotics that have been prescribed. Steam inhalation also helps relieve the congestion. If due to allergy, follow recommendations under allergic rhinitis.

Notes: ⎯⎯⎯⎯⎯⎯⎯⎯⎯⎯⎯⎯⎯⎯⎯⎯⎯⎯⎯⎯⎯⎯⎯⎯⎯⎯⎯

Accupressure, accupuncture are other forms of treatment. In chronic cases, surgery may be done. In mild cases, it is treated symptomatically.

Sleep Apnea

Respiratory system

A condition where there is stoppage of breathing for 10 seconds or longer, 30 times or more during a 7 hour sleeping period.

Cause:

The cause may be due to abnormalities in the respiratory center of the brain that controls the respiratory rate and depth (central sleep apnea) or due to obstruction to the air flow in the mouth or pharynx while sleeping (obstructive sleep apnea). In some individuals it may be due to both reasons (mixed sleep apnea).

Signs and Symptoms:

Noisy snoring, difficulty in falling asleep (insomnia), sleepiness during the day, abnormal movements during sleep are some of the symptoms. It may be associated with early morning headaches and psychological problems like sexual impotence and depression.

Risk factors:

Encephalitis, poliomyelitis affecting the brain stem can predispose to central sleep apnea. Obstructive type is commoner in middle-aged men and obese individuals. Alcohol and drugs that depress the central nervous system also predispose to obstructive sleep apnea.

Caution and Recommendations to Therapists:

Encourage clients to loose weight. Sleeping on the side instead of the back helps reduce obstructive type of apnea. Massage is not contraindicated in this condition. It helps relax these tired and depressed individuals.

Notes: ————————————————————————————

Sleep apnea is treated in many ways according to the cause. While sleeping, nasal masks that literally push the air into the respiratory tract are sometimes used. Drugs are also used to stimulate the respiratory center. Rarely, surgery is done to correct the nasal passage if the cause is due to abnormal nasal septum.

Spina bifida (Meningocele, Myelomenigocele)

Nervous system

A defect in the fusion of the right and left half of one or more vertebrae during the development of the foetus resulting in malformation of the spine. There may or may not be protrusion of the spinal cord and meninges through the gap.

Cause:

Virus infection, exposure to radiation or other toxic environmental factors during the first three months of pregnancy - when the spinal cord and vertebrae develop, can produce malformation of the spine. Usually the defect is in the lower back -

lumbosacral region.

Signs and Symptoms:

In spina bifida occulta - the commonest and least severe form, there is a depression, tuft of hair, birth mark or soft fatty tissue on the skin over the region. It may be asymptomatic or associated with weakness of the legs, urinary bladder or bowel dysfunction. In the more severe defect, the meninges and cerebro spinal fluid (CSF) protrude out (meningocele) or there is protrusion of the spinal cord along with the meninges and CSF (myelomeningocele), producing a sac like appearance in the region. The severe forms are accompanied by weakness or paralysis of the legs. There may be associated hydrocephalus and mental retardation.

Risk factors:

There is a genetic predisposition. Exposure to radiation, Rubella or other viral infections early in pregnancy also produce this condition.

Caution and Recommendations to Therapists:

In the less severe form avoid massaging the lumbosacral area. In the more severe form with neurological problems, the aim is to prevent contractures, pressure ulcers and reduce spasticity. Passive movements and range of motion exercises of joints prevent contractures of muscles. Use transverse friction strokes around joints. Do not use force to stretch muscles that are in spasm. These individuals are prone for decubitus (pressure) ulcers and edema in the dependent parts such as the legs or sacral region. The poor circulation in these areas makes the skin very fragile with a tendency to breakdown with minimal pressure. Avoid massaging areas with ulcers and bring it to the notice of the caregivers. Some clients may also have reduced sensations. Use mild to moderate pressure in these areas. Refer client to local support groups (see Appendix IV).

Notes: ───

Spina bifida occulta is not treated medically. The more severe forms are treated by surgery. Crutches, braces are used to help those with neurological dysfunctions.

Spinal cord injury Nervous system

Complete or partial damage to the spinal cord at any level resulting in loss of sensation, motor function and autonomic function.

Cause:

Trauma is the commonest cause. The problems that result is not only due to the direct damage but also to the reaction of the body to the injury in the form of edema, bleeding, reduced blood supply and inflammation of the cord. Other causes include tumors.

Signs and Symptoms:

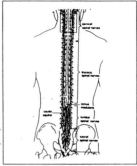

Within the first twenty four hours the person looses all function below the level of injury - spinal shock. In spinal shock, sensations, motor activity as well as autonomic function is lost. In due course the functions resume depending on the extent and site of damage.

If the whole cord is cut, there is complete loss of sensations and motor function below the level of injury. If the injury is at the cervical region quadriplegia (paralysis of all four limbs) results. If above C4, the nerve supply to the diaphragm is affected and the person requires mechanical ventilation. If below, paraplegia (paralysis of the lower limbs) results with or without involvement of the trunk muscles. Injury at the thoracic level affects the nerve supply to the intercostal muscles and impairs respiration making the person prone to respiratory infection.

The muscles are spastic (increased in tone) and the reflexes are exaggerated. The muscles have a tendency to get fixed in a flexed position. The lack of muscle tone makes the person prone to edema. Pressure ulcers are common due to lack of sensation and abnormal autonomic function. Bladder and bowel control are lost. The absence of stress on the bones supporting the paralyzed muscles, causes osteoporosis. The absorption of calcium from the bone and excretion through the kidneys, along with the stagnation of urine in the bladder make the person prone for stone formation in the kidneys and urinary tract infection. The absence of movement around the veins of the limbs also make them prone for deep vein thrombosis. Lesions above the level of T6 can result in abnormal autonomic reflexes such as sudden increase in blood pressure, flushing, increased sweating and headache on even mild stimulation below the level of lesion. The lack of autonomic control affects the regulation of temperature and blood pressure.

Risk factors:

The most common cause is motor vehicle accidents.

Caution and Recommendations to Therapists:

Assessment of the client before massage is very important. Keep a record of the extent of the loss of function - both sensory and motor. The aim is to reduce spasticity, improve circulation; prevent edema and pressure ulcers, prevent contractures and maintain the range of motion in joints. Caution is required as the sensations are impaired and proper feedback may not be forthcoming. Also they are prone for deep vein thrombosis. Dislodgment of thrombus can cause further complications.

Position the client in a neutral position with the legs in line with the rest of body. A number of cushions may be required. Elevate the limbs with cushions if edema is present even before beginning treatment. Keep the client warm. Use lymphatic drainage techniques to help reduce edema. Watch for pressure ulcers and avoid areas of ulcers leaving a wide margin around it. Use gentle rhythmic and repetitive strokes in general. However, stimulatory massage to the extensor muscles can reduce the tone in the flexors which are more hypertonic than extensors. Use tapotement and vibration strokes over chest wall to help drain the mucus. The head end can be lowered while massaging the chest as this uses the effect of gravity for drainage.

Give sufficient support when the position of the client is changed as they are prone for postural hypotension. Involuntary spasms and movements are common in these clients so do not be alarmed. Passively move the joints through as wide a range of motion without using force. Transverse friction should be used around joints to prevent adhesions and contractures. Concentrate also on muscles that are excessively stressed by compensatory overuse. Massage is indicated on an ongoing basis. Schedule once or twice a week and modify the duration according to individuals.

Notes: ————————————————————————————————————

Sprain Musculoskeletal system

A complete or incomplete tear in the ligament/s around a joint. There is no displacement of or instability to the joint.

Cause:

It follows a sudden, sharp twist to the joint that stretches the ligament and ruptures some or all of the fibres.

Signs and Symptoms:

There is local pain, especially during joint movement, swelling, loss of mobility and discoloration of the skin over the joint due to the extravasation of blood into the surrounding tissues from the injured ligament. Sprains occur more commonly in the ankle, wrist and back. The client usually gives a history of recent injury or prolonged overuse.

Risk factors:

Occupations and sports that require use of ankles and wrists extensively have a high risk of causing sprain.

Caution and Recommendations to Therapists:

In acute cases, use icepack intermittently to reduce pain and swelling. The joint should be elevated above the heart to use the effect of gravity to reduce edema. The joint is immobilized for 1-3 weeks depending on the extent of the rupture. Passively move joints that are not affected. Massage adjacent muscles to increase circulation, reduce swelling and address trigger points. The aim of massage at the time of healing is to prevent adhesions. Deep transverse friction that move the ligaments over the bone are advocated. Deep moist heat helps soften scar tissue and increase circulation.

Notes: ────────────────────────────────

Sprains are classified as mild, moderate or severe according to the extent of injury to the ligaments.

═══

Sprain - ankle (Anterior talofibular or Calcaneocuboid ligament injury)
Musculoskeletal system

Partial or complete tear of one of the ligaments in the ankle.

Cause:

A forced stress on the ankle usually produces this condition. It is the most commonly sprained area in the body. Typically, it is seen in athletes who jump and land on the lateral border of the foot that has been plantar flexed, or by excessive inversion of the foot as when a high heel gets caught on uneven ground.

Signs and Symptoms:

It presents as pain over the ankle and/or pain referred distally or proximally. The severity of the pain does not correspond to the extent of injury. Mild or moderate injury produces more pain than a complete tear. There may be discoloration in the area due to the extravasation of blood. In acute cases, movement is painful and restricted due to effusion of fluid in the joint and muscle spasm. In chronic cases, passive foot movement is painless and hypermobility may be seen if there is complete rupture. In chronic, recurrent injuries, the sprain presents as sudden giving way of the ankle. This may be followed by swelling and pain for a few days.

Risk factors:

It is common in active young individuals who are engaged in sports that involve jumping.

Caution and Recommendations to Therapists:

In acute cases, ice application and elevation of foot is recommended. To aid the healing process rest is advised. However, active movement should be encouraged to prevent stiffness and muscle atrophy. Passively move the joint in a direction that does not stress the ligament. Friction massage may be used in the subacute stage to prevent adhesions. It should be noted that although collagen fibres are laid down within the first few weeks it takes months for the collagen to mature, realign and regain original strength (see under Sprain for further details).

Notes: _____

Sprain - knee   Musculoskeletal system

A complete or incomplete tear of the ligaments around the knee joint.

Cause:

It is usually caused by trauma to the knee. It is a common injury in football players while being tackled from the side. The sudden force from the side on the slightly flexed knee and planted foot produces forward movement of the femur and external rotation of the tibia resulting in tear in the medial collateral ligament and /or capsule and medial meniscus. The anterior cruciate ligament can be torn by forward forces on an extended or near extended thigh. The posterior cruciate ligament is stretched by a sudden backward movement of the tibia on the femur.

Signs and Symptoms:

The pain is localized to the site of the tear. There is joint swelling with synovial

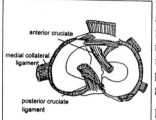

fluid or blood. The pain may be referred to the L3, L4 and S2 segment as nerves supplying the knee arise from here. Thus, pain may be felt in the lower lumbar region, front and back of thigh or back of calf. The pain is increased by moving the knee in directions that produce stress on the ligament. There is muscle guarding in the acute stage.

In chronic sprains, the client complains of giving way of the knee. There is also difficulty in performing specific activities like squatting, turning sharply or going down the stairs. There is associated atrophy of the quadriceps muscle and hypermobility of the joint.

Risk factors:

Sprain of the knee is common in young active individuals.

Caution and Recommendations to Therapists:

Assess the joint to see if the sprain is mild - Grade I (very little loss of integrity of ligament, not hypermobile), moderate - Grade II (mild hypermobility) or severe - Grade III (marked hypermobility). In mild to moderate injury, use icepacks if acute. In the subacute or chronic stage transverse friction massage is used - in a direction perpendicular to the line of ligament with the knee flexed at different degrees. This prevents adhesion to adjacent structures and also helps align the newly formed collagen fibres. For grade III sprains the limb is immobilized with cast. Massage muscles around cast to improve circulation. After removal of cast use transverse friction massage around the joint. Encourage client to do remedial exercises to maintain and improve range of motion. Always work in conjunction with a physiotherapist (see under Sprains for more details).

Half hour schedules two to three times a week for the first few weeks are recommended.

Notes: ───

The normal knee is capable of flexing 130-150 degrees, extending 0-3 degrees, and rotating internally or externally by 10 degrees.

Still's disease (Juvenile Rheumatoid Arthritis)
Musculoskeletal system

An autoimmune disease that affects multiple systems in children, producing degenerative changes in connective tissue and inflammatory vascular lesions.

Cause:

It is due to the immune system of the body reacting to tissues of self as it would to foreign tissues.

Signs and Symptoms:

The symptoms are similar to that of rheumatoid arthritis in adults (see Arthritis - rheumatoid). The spleen and lymph nodes are also enlarged.

Risk factors:

It affects children under 16 years of age and is more common in females. Viral or bacterial infections, emotional stress and trauma have been known to precipitate the disease.

Caution and Recommendations to Therapists:

See Arthritis - rheumatoid.

Notes: _____

Stomatitis

Gastrointestinal system

An inflammation of the mucosa of the mouth.

Cause:

Stomatitis may be due to various factors. Herpes stomatitis is due to Herpes Simplex virus infection (see under Herpes Simplex). The cause of Aphthous stomatitis is unknown. Allergic stomatitis is due to hypersensitivity to food or lipstick. Thrush is another form of stomatitis caused by yeast infection.

Signs and Symptoms:

In the type due to Herpes, the person also has systemic symptoms of fever, irritability, loss of appetite along with pain in the mouth. The submaxillary lymph glands may be enlarged and painful. In the aphthous type, single or multiple shallow ulcers may be seen on the mucosa of the mouth, palate or lip. In thrush, patchy ulcers covered by a white cheesy material are seen in the mouth and pharynx (see under Thrush).

Risk factors:

Herpes Simplex infection in other areas may spread to this region. Aphthous Stomatitis can be predisposed by stress, fatigue, anxiety, trauma, sunburn, hypersensitivity to drugs or food, or other systemic diseases.

Caution and Recommendations to Therapists:

Stomatitis due to Herpes can spread to other areas in the person as well as to others on contact. Do not massage till completely treated.

In other types, avoid massaging face and neck if the lymph nodes are enlarged and inflamed.

Notes: ───────────────────────────────

Both types of stomatitis heal spontaneously. Antiseptic mouth washes should not be used as it is irritable to the inflamed area. The stomatitis heals in 10-14 days.

═══

Strain   Musculoskeletal system

A stretching injury to a muscle that results in partial or complete tear.

Cause:

Strains are usually caused by acute or chronic mechanical overloading.

Signs and Symptoms:

Pain, swelling and stiffness is seen in the affected area. Sometimes a snapping sound may be heard followed by rapid swelling soon after the injury. The muscle is tender and pain is increased on actively contracting or passively stretching the muscle. A few days later ecchymoses (small spots of bleeding under the skin) may be seen. If the strain is mild there is muscle spasm and tenderness over the region. There may be slight weakness of muscle. In moderate strain, along with more severe symptoms of mild strain, bruising may be seen. In severe strain, the function of muscle is lost, with excruciating pain if the muscle is not fully ruptured. If fully ruptured there may be no pain associated.

Strain is more common in the lower back and neck. In the hip the hamstrings, adductor longus, iliopsoas and rectus femoris are the most commonly strained muscles.

Risk factors:

Overweight, strenuous exercises and poor posture are the commonest predisposing factors. Abnormal strength ratios of agonist and antagonist muscles as seen in weight trainers who concentrate on strengthening only one group of muscles, increases the risk of strain.

Caution and Recommendations for Therapists:

Use cold applications during the first 24-48 hours to reduce pain and swelling. The unaffected areas should be massaged to reduce muscle spasm and thereby lessen pain. Avoid massaging distal to the site of injury. Passively move all joints adjacent to the injury to maintain range of movement. Care should be taken not to stretch the injured muscle.

In the subacute stage, techniques to reduce swelling should be employed. Later transverse friction massage is used to prevent formation of adhesions, and random alignment of the newly laid collagen fibres. Use gentle stretching manipulations. Refer to physiotherapist for strengthening exercises.

Initially, half hour treatments, once or twice a week is recommended. The frequency can be reduced according to the progress of the condition.

Note: _____

Stroke (Cerebrovascular accident, CVA)   Nervous system

A sudden reduction of blood supply to areas of the brain.

Cause:

The reduction in blood supply is due to either thrombosis/embolism which block the blood vessel, or hemorrhage. This results in reduced oxygen supply to the brain tissue. The hypoxia (reduced oxygen) causes congestion and edema of the brain. The latter produce the symptoms and signs associated with stroke. If the lack of oxygen supply lasts for a few minutes irreversible damage is done to the brain tissue.

Signs and Symptoms:

This varies with the artery that is affected and the duration of lack of blood supply and the ability of the surrounding arteries to compensate for the lack of blood supply to the area. If the left side of the brain is affected the symptoms are seen on the right side and vice versa. Some of the associated signs and symptoms seen are difficulty in speech, weakness of muscles in one side of the body with certain groups of muscles more affected than the others (hemiplegia), complete or partial loss of sight. There may also be accompanying loss or decrease in sensations. Poor coordination, abnormalities in their gait are other signs that may be present.

Disorientation, headache, convulsions, coma are other general symptoms. Autonomic problems like constipation may be present.

As a massage therapist, one may come in contact with clients who are in the recovery or rehabilitatory phase of stroke where the muscles are weak, spastic (rigid), with reflexes that are exaggerated. In these individuals, typically, the arm is held adducted with elbows partly flexed and pronated, and fingers flexed. The legs are extended with the foot plantar flexed. The facial muscles may or may not be affected with the cheeks lax and lip depressed on one side. The eyelids may droop on one side. Sensation may be altered and tremors of one of the limbs may be present. In clients with long term paralysis, skin changes and contractures may also be seen. It may be accompanied by depression, lack of concentration and memory loss.

Risk factors:

History of transient ischemic attacks, atherosclerosis, hypertension, postural hypotension, cerebral aneurysms, cardiac arrhythmias, diabetes mellitus, high cholesterol levels are high risk factors. A sedentary lifestyle, smoking, family history of cerebro vascular accidents and use of contraceptives are other predisposing factors.

Caution and Recommendations to Therapists:

The aim is to prevent joint stiffness and deformity, decrease spasticity, re-educate the perception of sensory stimuli and movement patterns, reduce skin changes and edema and address postural changes like scoliosis and kyphosis that may occur due to the weakness of muscles. Work in conjunction with a physiotherapist and occupational therapist.

Spend time to assess the sensory and motor functions and keep a good record of your findings in order to individualize treatment and track progress of the client. For assessing motor function, test the range of motion possible in all joints. Note the level of spasticity. Spasticity is the resistance offered to a particular movement when the joint is passively moved. Careful assessment of the factors that precipitate a spasm in the client should be obtained. Stretching of muscles, pressure or irritation of the skin are some of the common stimuli for spasm. For assessment of sensory function, ask clients about decreased or loss of sensation in specific areas. These areas may be tested for perception to light touch - as with stroking with a feather, and for temperature and pain perception - by using warm and cold water in a small container. Also look for skin changes and pressure ulcers. The pressure used during massage, and use of hydrotherapy should be modified according to the findings.

Position the client with the spine and neck straight and the shoulder and pelvis aligned over each other. Cover the parts that are not being worked on making sure that the client is kept warm.

All the affected joints should be moved passively through the full range of movement possible. Do not forcibly move spastic muscles. To help re-educate the limb ask the client to perform the same movement using the unaffected side. Stimulate the muscles antagonistic to the spastic muscles using tapotement. This can help reduce the spasticity eg. stimulating the triceps can reduce spasticity in the biceps muscle.

The massage strokes should be slow and superficial, soothing and rhythmic. Excessive stimulation may increase the spasticity. Clonus - abnormal involuntary movements with alternate contraction and relaxation especially of the ankle joint is normal in these clients. This is seen if the ankle is dorsiflexed suddenly. Do not be alarmed if clonus is present. Adjust pressure according to each client. The skin is fragile and easily damaged on the affected side. In addition, the sensation may be altered and the feed back from the client may be inadequate. Closely monitor the temperature of heating pads (if used) due to the reduced sensation in these clients. Massage the unaffected side - especially those areas that are overused. Encourage clients to use both affected and unaffected side.

In the case of treating clients in the early stages -within a week or two, the muscles may be flaccid - with reduced tone. In such cases, use friction, effleurage and petrissage as such strokes have been shown to increase muscle tone.

The first few treatments should be short - not more than half an hour, once or twice a week. This should be slowly increased to durations of one hour.

Refer clients to local support groups. See Appendix IV for resources.

Notes: ─────────────────────────────

Regular aerobic and/or stretch exercises are helpful. Alternative therapy include yoga, tai chi, meditation and imagery.

Synovitis - acute   Musculoskeletal system

An acute inflammation of the lining membrane of joints.

Cause:

It usually follows any form of injury to the joint. Some inflammation of the synovial membrane is present in any type of arthritis.

Signs and Symptoms:

The joint shows sign of inflammation - redness, heat, swelling, pain and loss of function. The skin may be reddened if the inflammation has spread. The joint is swollen due to the movement of fluid into it. A dull and aching pain is present at rest. The pain increases on moving the joint. To minimize pain the client keeps the limb in a position that relaxes the ligaments around the joint. Atrophy of the muscles around the joint may be seen in those with prolonged inflammation.

Risk factors:

See Cause.

Caution and Recommendations to Therapists:

Care of the client should be directed towards preventing the spread of inflammation, relief of pain, reduction of swelling and assisting with the reabsorption of fluid and toxins thereby preventing adhesions. The aim should also be to prevent disuse atrophy of muscles and to help client regain joint range and function.

The limb should be well supported with pillows. During the first 24 hours, cold application gives relief. Cold packs or towels immersed in cold water and then wrung out can be applied over area.

During the first few days mild heat helps reduce swelling and pain. In acute synovitis the client may be unable to tolerate much manipulation. Light squeezing movements in an upward direction with each hand on the side of the limb may help. Gentle effleurage can be substituted according to the tolerance of the individual. Gentle finger kneading may be added over the joint to reduce the swelling and prevent adhesions. To maintain circulation, the parts of the limb that can be reached without moving the affected joint should be massaged vigorously.

When the inflammation has subsided and there is no pain, deep friction around the affected joint should be resorted to along with heat application. Passive movement also helps. Encourage client to exercise the joint at this stage.

Notes: ————————————————————————————

Synovitis - chronic   Musculoskeletal system

A chronic inflammation of the lining membrane of joints.

Cause:

It can be caused by repeated acute synovitis, recurrent injuries or strains to the joint. Loose bodies like broken bones, bits of cartilage inside the joint or abnormal alignment of the articulating surfaces joint can also result in this chronic problem.

Signs and Symptoms:

Chronic synovitis is characterized by thickening of the synovial membrane and long-standing swelling of the joint. The muscles around the joint are atrophied and the joint tends to buckle due to the lax and stretched ligaments. There may be a dull aching pain and stiffness of the joint.

Risk factors:

See risk factors for Synovitis - acute.

Caution and Recommendations to Therapists:

Any form of heat is soothing. Use kneading and deep friction strokes over and around the joint. Passive movements of the joints also help break up adhesions.

Notes: _____

Syphilis

Reproductive, Integumentary systems

A chronic, infectious, sexually transmitted disease.

Cause:

It is caused by the bacteria Treponema pallidum. It is transmitted by intimate physical contact. The bacteria enters the mucous membrane and spreads to the local lymph nodes and then to the blood stream producing systemic symptoms. It can spread to the fetus from infected mothers. The incubation period lasts for about 3 weeks.

Signs and Symptoms:

Typically, it presents as painless, fluid-filled lesions in the genitalia and other regions of contact such as the mouth, tongue, nipples etc. These lesions (chancres) are firm to touch with raised edges. The local lymph nodes may be enlarged. The chancres may disappear within 3-6 weeks with or without treatment. If untreated, generalized lymph node enlargement and skin rashes occur within 8 weeks after the onset of chancres. These rashes are highly contagious.

The late stage of syphilis (very rare after the availability of antibiotics) which occurs 1-10 years after infection is noninfectious. But it is destructive and affects many systems.

Risk factors:

The incidence is higher in urban regions, in drug users and those with AIDS.

Caution and Recommendations to Therapists:

Massage is contraindicated. Encourage clients with painless fluid filled lesions around the mouth, tongue etc. to seek medical help.

Notes: _____

Systemic Lupus Erythematosus (SLE)

Cardiovascular, Musculoskeletal, Integumentary, Renal, Pulmonary systems

A chronic autoimmune inflammatory disease.

Cause:

The cause is unknown. It is considered to be autoimmune as there is production of autoantibodies and immune complexes that affect multiple systems.

Signs and Symptoms:

It is called "the great imitator" as the signs and symptoms resemble that of many other diseases. The onset may be acute or chronic and there is exacerbation and remission of the disease. Most clients present with joint pain. Chronic inflammation of the joint makes the ligaments, tendons and capsule lax and susceptible to deformities. In the acute form of SLE, a butterfly shaped rash is seen over the nose and cheek (see Appendix I figure 12). Glomerulonephritis (inflammation in the kidney), pulmonary effusion (fluid collection in the lungs), pericarditis (inflammation of the membrane surrounding the heart) are some of the other manifestations. The client may also have central nervous system effects such as psychosis, depression, confusion and dementia. Lymph node enlargement may be seen in some.

Risk factors:

It is more common in females especially in the child bearing age group. Estrogens favor the development of the disease while androgens protect. African-Americans and Asians are at less risk. There is also a genetic predisposition. SLE can be triggered by ultra-violet light, chemicals such as hair dyes, drugs, certain types of food and infectious agents.

Caution and Recommendations to Therapists:

Clients may be on corticosteroids and anti-inflammatory drugs. Some may also be on other drugs that suppress immunity. Care should be taken to minimize exposure of such clients to any form of infection. A whole body relaxation massage is indicated. Avoid areas that are acutely inflamed. Special care of joints such as passive movements, friction to reduce adhesions are required for those with chronic arthritis. Application of warm packs may be beneficial. Refer client to support groups (see Appendix IV).

Notes: _____

Temporomandibular joint dysfunction syndrome (Mandibular pain dysfunction syndrome, Arthrosis temporo mandibularis, Temporo mandibular joint arthrosis, Myofascial pain syndrome)

Musculoskeletal system

A collection of symptoms and signs produced by temporomandibular joint disorders.

Cause:

It is caused by inappropriate alignment of the joint and/or laxity of the supporting ligaments and muscle. There may be degenerative changes in the joint.

Signs and Symptoms:

This syndrome is characterized by unilateral or bilateral muscle tenderness and reduced motion. There is a dull aching pain around the joint, often radiating to the ear, face, neck or shoulder. The syndrome may start off as clicking sounds in the joint. There may be protrusion of the jaw or hypermobility on opening the jaw accompanied by pain. Slowly it progresses to decreased mobility of the jaw. Locking of the jaw may occur. If the problem is unilateral, the jaw may deviate to the side affected with resultant hypermobility and subluxation (loss of alignment) of the other jaw.

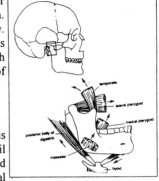

Risk factors:

It is more common between 20-40 years of age and is more frequently seen in women. Gum chewing, nail biting, mouth breathing, prolonged use of pacifiers and bottles, biting off large chunks of hard food, habitual protrusion of jaws, stress translated into tension of muscles of neck and back and clenching of jaw, predispose to this condition. Injury/ trauma, whiplash injuries, improper braces are other risk factors. In some people a genetic predisposition have been identified. Rarely, rheumatoid arthritis may affect this joint.

Caution and Recommendations to Therapists:

It is important to assess and palpate the specific muscles both intra and extra orally. Ensure that latex gloves are worn while palpating intra orally. The masseters, temporalis muscle and pterygoids both medial and lateral should be palpated for spasm, tenderness and trigger points. The range and symmetry of movement of the jaw should also be tested.

The aim of treatment is to reduce the pain and spasm of muscles and to relax and strengthen the muscles involved. The cause has to be identified in order to produce long term improvement.

In the acute stage, hot packs can be used to relieve muscle pain and spasm. Ice packs can be used if inflammation of the joint is present. The muscles of the neck, occiput and shoulders have to be thoroughly massaged to reduce spasm and trigger points.

Later soft tissue mobilization techniques are employed. Deep friction massage is given to the capsule of the joint. Gentle stroking or kneading at the insertion of the temporalis and medial and lateral pterygoids intra-orally may also used. Myofascial release techniques help relax the muscles of mastication such as the masseter, temporalis, supra and infra hyoid muscles. Mobilization techniques like caudal traction, protrusion, medial-lateral glide can be used.

The client has to be educated to relax the muscles. This can be done by asking the client to clench the jaw firmly and concentrate on the sense and feeling of tightness of jaw. Then he/she is asked to relax and let the jaw fall open. Alternately, the jaw is opened against resistance provided by the therapist, followed by total relaxation. Other movements to the right and left are also performed with and without resistance and then allowed to relax. The client can also be advised on maintaining proper posture and breathing techniques. Passive and active stretches are other forms of treatment used. Consult dentist and physiotherapist for specific treatment techniques.

Ensure that the client does not harbor any infective disease that can be transmitted by secretions, at the time of treatment. Always use disposable latex gloves while manipulating intra orally.

Notes: ———————————————————————————————

Special skills are required to massage the muscles involved and training is required to asses the joint and perform the massage techniques correctly.

Tendinitis - Achilles   Musculoskeletal system

Inflammation of the Achilles tendon (tendo calcaneus).

Cause:

It is caused by overuse of the gastrocnemius and soleus muscles.

Signs and Symptoms:

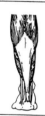

There is gradual onset of pain behind the ankle, that increases on inverting, everting or dorsiflexing the foot. The pain may be in areas proximal to the insertion of the tendon to the calcaneus ie. at the region with the poorest blood supply.

The pain may also be associated with inflammation of the infratendinous and supratendinous bursa. There may be swelling of the tendon. Crepitations (abnormal crackling sounds) may be heard on moving the ankle in the case of inflammation of the connective tissue around the Achilles.

Risk factors:

High impact sports such as basketball, running, volleyball predispose to this condition.

Caution and Recommendations to Therapists:

In the acute state, the part should be rested. Ice, compression and elevation of the limb are used to minimize swelling. Later, deep transverse friction massage is used. (see tendinitis-supraspinatus for friction massage techniques)

Notes: ─────────────────────────────────────

Tendinitis - bicipital   Musculoskeletal system

Inflammation of the tendon of the biceps near its insertion.

Cause:

It is commonly caused by acute trauma to the elbow or recurrent overuse. Other musculoskeletal disorders such as rheumatic diseases, congenital defects, postural misalignment or hypermobility may also cause this.

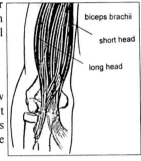

biceps brachii

short head

long head

Signs and Symptoms:

There is a gradual onset of pain in the front of the elbow radiating down the forearm. Painful twinges are also felt when the elbow is flexed or supinated.Biceps tendinitis can be recognized by the pain produced on extending the elbow with the shoulder extended.

Risk factors:

Activities that involve recurrent flexion of the elbow or supination of the forearm predispose to this condition.

Caution and Recommendations to Therapists:

In acute cases, ice application and restriction of movement is beneficial. However, joints should be moved gently to minimize loss of extensibility of the muscle and tendon and to prevent stiffening. Such a treatment should be continued for 3-4 days.

In chronic cases, strong repetitive movements should be restricted as long as pain persists. Heat therapy can help reduce pain. Start with gentle effleurage and kneading strokes and later, use deep transverse friction (See Tendinitis - supraspinatus for details of transverse friction technique). Transverse friction promotes proper orientation of the fibres along line of stress without causing additional trauma to the healing tendon. Later, add stretches to the line of treatment by extending elbow with the forearm pronated. Exercises to strengthen the atrophied muscles should be added last. Clients on anti-inflammatory therapy will have a higher threshold for pain and there are chances of overtreating the client inadvertently.

Notes: _____

Tendinitis - elbow (Tennis elbow, Epitrochlear bursitis, Golfer's elbow)

Musculoskeletal system

Inflammation of the origin/insertion of muscles and tendons around the elbow.

Cause:

It is due due to overstrain of muscles while playing tennis or other activities that

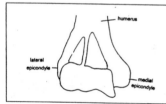

involve forceful grasp, extension of wrist against resistance, or repeated rotation of the forearm. Lateral tennis elbow involves the origin of the extensor carpi radialis brevis, or the common aponeurosis of the extensors at the lateral epicondyle. Medial epicondylitis or golfers elbow involves the inflammation of the flexor tendons as they arise from the medial epicondyle. Posterior tennis elbow is rare and involves the inflammation of the triceps tendon.

Signs and Symptoms:

There is a gradual onset of pain in the elbow. The pain radiates to the back of the arm and wrist on grasping objects. Tenderness may be present over the lateral or medial epicondyle, or head of radius. Increased temperature, swelling and reduced range of motion may be seen during the acute phase. The grip may also be weaker.

Risk factors:

Occupations which involve overstrain of the muscles that originate - insert at the elbow increase the risk.

Caution and Recommendations to Therapists:

Assessment is done with the elbow extended and supported between the therapist's elbow and side, and with the clients forearm cradled on the forearm and hand. In lateral tennis elbow, pain or restricted movement is noted on wrist flexion, ulnar deviation with the forearm pronated and flexed. In medial tennis elbow, pain is felt when the wrist and fingers are fully extended and the forearm supinated.

In acute cases, ice application along with restriction of movements helps. However, the joints should be moved gently to minimize loss of extensibility of the muscle and tendon. Such a treatment should be continued for 3-4 days. Start with gentle effleurage and kneading strokes during the acute stage.

In chronic cases, strong repetitive movement should be restricted as long as pain persists. Heat therapy helps reduce pain. Passively move all joints to prevent stiffening. Use deep transverse friction over the tendon. Transverse friction promotes proper orientation of the fibres along line of stress without causing additional trauma to the healing tendon tissue. To access the tendon, the wrist is positioned fully flexed, with the elbow in semi-flexion, and the arm abducted and internally rotated. Follow the friction with ice massage.

Add stretches to the line of treatment. The muscles can be stretched by extending the elbow with the forearm pronated, wrist ulnar deviated and the wrist and fingers flexed. Exercises to strengthen the atrophied muscles should be added last. Clients on anti-inflammatory therapy will have a higher threshold for pain and there are chances of overtreating the client inadvertently.

Half hour treatments daily or three times a week followed by twice a week for one week and once a week for another two weeks are recommended.

Advice the client to refrain from activities that may cause tendinitis for 2-6 weeks or until healing has occurred.

Notes: ─────────────────────────────────────

Tendinitis - patellar (Jumper's knee)

Musculoskeletal system

Inflammation of the patellar or quadriceps tendon as it attaches to the tibial tuberosity and the patella.

Cause:

Overuse of the quadriceps muscle can cause this.

Signs and Symptoms:

There is pain over the knee along with swelling and joint tenderness. The pain increases on extension of the knee.

Risk factors:

The incidence is higher in occupations that involve repetitive extension of the leg. Sports activities like basketball or volleyball that require repetitive jumping can also predispose to this.

Caution and Recommendations to Therapists:

Ice massage reduces inflammation in the acute stage. Friction massage (see Tendinitis - supraspinatus for techniques) to the tendon is helpful once the inflammation has subsided. Stretching of the muscle and ice application should be given following friction. The spasm and trigger points in the proximal and antagonist muscles should be addressed as well. The range of motion of the knee joint should be maintained by passive movements.

Notes: _____

Tendinitis - popliteal/semi membranosus

Musculoskeletal system

Inflammation of the popliteal or semimembranosus tendon.

Cause:

It is caused by overuse of the muscles by repetitive flexion of the knee.

Signs and Symptoms:

Pain is felt over the lateral surface of the knee especially over the attachment of the muscle to the lateral surface of the femoral condyle.

Risk factors:

It is more common in long distance runners.

Caution and Recommendations to Therapists:

Advice the client to rest. Use ice massage for the first 72 hours. Follow up by stretches and passive movements. Friction around the joint is beneficial.

Use deep strokes to soften and stretch adhesions and scar tissue after the inflammation has subsided.

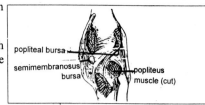

Notes: _____

Tendinitis - supraspinatous, infraspinatus

(Shoulder impingement syndrome)   Musculoskeletal system

Painful inflammation of the supraspinatus/infraspinatus tendon at the muscle-tendon attachment to the humerus.

Cause:

The supraspinatus tendon, being attached to the greater tuberosity of the humerus is prone to compression between the acromion of the scapula and the humerus when the arm is abducted and the humeral head slips under the acromion. Prolonged overuse causes thickening of the tendon and bone spur formation which increase the chances of compression. In addition, compared to other muscles of the rotator cuff, the supra and infraspinatus are less vascular and more prone to degenerative changes. Tendinitis is commonly caused by acute trauma to the shoulder or recurrent overuse. Other musculoskeletal disorders such as rheumatic diseases, congenital defects, postural misalignment or hypermobility can also result cause this.

Signs and Symptoms:

The client has restricted abduction of shoulder due to the compression of the inflamed and swollen tendon against the acromion. There is localized pain that presents as a sharp twinge on abducting the arm between 50 and 130 degree arc. The pain is often severe at night and is felt in the lateral aspect of the arm extending from the acromion to the insertion of the deltoid. There may be swelling due to fluid accumulation. A crepitus (crackling sound) may be felt over the site of the tendon.

Risk factors:

It is more common in young active individuals. Activities such as tennis, swimming, racquetball, and baseball which involve repeated elevation of arm to the level of the shoulder or above predispose this condition.

Caution and Recommendations to Therapists:

If the inflammation is acute, ice can be applied to reduce swelling and pain.

Transverse friction massage is an important component of treatment in chronic tendinitis. It mobilizes scar tissue that is forming or which has already developed and also increases blood flow to the area thus speeding up healing. Deep moist heat should be used to soften scars and adhesions before friction massage. For transverse friction massage to the shoulder, the client should be seated, the shoulder exposed completely, and the elbow supported to reduce muscle tension.

To access the supraspinatus tendon, the limb should be placed in adduction, and internal rotation, by asking the client to flex the elbow and keep the forearm close to the small of the back. The insertion can be felt near the acromion, on the highest impression of the greater tubercle of the humerus. To access the infraspinatus tendon, the arm should be flexed, adducted and laterally rotated. Such a position may be obtained by asking the client to lie prone, with the body resting on the elbow of the laterally rotated limb.

Without lubricant, use pad of index finger, middle finger or thumb over the tendon which is between the acromion and the greater tuberosity of humerus, and apply light pressure. Move the skin over the site forward and backward, two to three times per second for 1-2 minutes, in a direction that is perpendicular to the direction of fibres in the tendon (ie. for the supraspinatus tendon, move in an antero-posterior direction). Even if tenderness is felt initially, it should disappear or reduce. If tenderness increases, stop treatment.

Skin blisters may develop if improper techniques (which increase friction between skin and the massaging finger) are used. To reduce friction, gather and support the skin over the shoulder with the thumb and fingers of the opposite hand. Do not do friction massage over skin of clients with already poor blood circulation. Such a condition is seen in clients on long-term corticosteroids or with peripheral vascular disease.

Passive movement of the arm within the limits of pain should also be employed. Work in close conjunction with the physiotherapist. Encourage client to do remedial strengthening exercises. Increase duration of treatment from 5-6 minutes in the first treatment to a maximum of 12-15 minutes. Usually a maximum of 6-10 sessions over 2-3 weeks are required for resolution. It is common for increased soreness to be felt after the first or secondsection. Ensure that the treatment is given over the lesion and not in the site of the pain. The latter may be referred to

266

a different site.

Therapists should take care not to overstress the distal interphalangeal joints while massaging. This can be avoided by supporting the massaging finger as well as by alternating different fingers for treatment.

Notes: _____

Tenosynovitis (Stenosing tenovaginitis, Hoffman's Disease)
Musculoskeletal system

Inflammation of the synovial sheath of muscles.

Cause:

It is caused by overwork of muscle, stretching or wrenching of a tendon or spread of inflammation from surrounding tissues. In injuries that break the skin and expose the tissue to the exterior, bacterial infection may cause this.

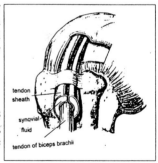

Signs and Symptoms:

There is swelling in the affected sheath with tenderness and pain on using the muscles. Crepitus (crackling sounds) may be produced by the friction between the roughened sheath of the tendon.

Risk factors:

Overwork of individual muscles predispose to this condition.

Caution and Recommendations to Therapists:

The aim is to smooth the roughened walls of the sheath and tendon and to free the tissues from adhesions. Deep transverse frictions should be used across the affected tendon. Keep the tendon stretched while massaging. Hot packs may help relieve pain. Regular massage over three months may be required. Half hourly treatment twice weekly is recommended.

Notes:

Synovial sheaths are synovial fluid filled sacs that are seen around certain tendons. It functions as a cushion that reduces friction between tendons and between bone and tendon.

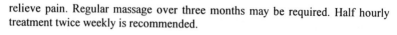

Tenosynovitis - bacterial

Musculoskeletal system

An inflammation in the synovial sheath of muscle, due to infection.

Cause:

Injuries that break skin and allow the entry of bacteria into the area cause this. The effects are particularly severe if it affects the thumb or fingers as it can spread all along the common synovial sheath up to the wrist. The flexor pollicis longus tendon has a long sheath from 2 inches proximal to the wrist to its insertion. The flexor sheath of the little finger is common with the sheath of the flexor profundus and sublimus. The sheaths of the middle fingers are unconnected with the common sheath.

Signs and Symptoms:

Pain, swelling and redness is seen along the length of the affected sheath. General symptoms such as fever is also seen. If pus has formed it may break through and spread to the surrounding tissues. It heals by fibrosis causing adhesions between adjacent structures and compromising the mobility. There may be generalized symptoms of fever, fatigue and loss of appetite.

Risk factors:

Any injury close to the sheath increases the risk.

Caution and Recommendations to Therapists:

In the acute stages refer to physician. The client may require surgery to release the

268

pus. Antibiotic treatment is also required. Do not massage until the infection has been treated completely.

In the chronic stage, deep effleurage, finger kneading and deep friction are required to release adhesions. Joints are often kept immobilized by the client due to the pain and this leads to stiffness of joints. Passive movement help mobilize the stiff joints. Use olive oil while massaging to soften the tissues. Improvement is very slow in this condition.

Notes: _____

Tenovaginitis - De Quervain's

Inflammation and swelling of the synovial lining of the common sheath of the abductor pollicis longus and extensor pollicis brevis as the tendons pass over the distal end of the radius.

Cause:

It is usually caused by trauma to the area.

Signs and Symptoms:

There is a slow onset of pain over the radius that may radiate to the thumb or proximally to the forearm. This pain is more on abducting or extending thumb as in performing wringing or grasping movements. There is tenderness over the tendon sheath as it passes over the styloid process of the radius. A spindle shaped thickening 2-3 inches long is felt over the distal end of the radius.

Risk factors:

Occupations involving repeated abduction and extension of thumb can predispose to this condition.

Caution and Recommendations to Therapists:

Assess by stretching the sheath. Pain is present on deviating the wrist towards the ulna while keeping the thumb flexed. When acute, use ice to reduce pain and swelling. When the inflammation has subsided, deep transverse friction is used at the rate of 3-5 times per week for one to two weeks. (See tendinitis - supraspinatus, for details of transverse friction technique). Transverse friction helps to resolve the inflammatory process and increase the mobility of the tendon within the sheath. Regular massage over a period of three months may be required. Half-hourly massage, twice weekly is recommended. The client should be advised not to overly exert the hand during the period of therapy.

Notes: _____

Tetanus

A bacterial neurological disorder characterized by increased muscle tone and spasms.

Cause:

It is caused by the toxin tetanospasmin released by the bacteria Clostridium tetani. The organism and its spores are found worldwide in soil, animal and sometimes human feces. The spores can survive for years and are resistant to various disinfectants and even boiling water for 20 minutes. However, the organisms are killed by antibiotics.

The organism enters through a contaminated wound and produces the toxin. Since it does not require oxygen for survival, it thrives in dead tissue, wounds contaminated with foreign bodies and active infection. The toxin released by the organism enters the motor neuron in the area and migrates through the axon, across synapses to reach the spinal cord and brain stem where it blocks the release of certain neurotransmitters that normally inhibit the impulses in the motor neuron. As a result, the motor neuron fires more than usual causing rigidity in the muscles. The toxin also affects the sympathetic system increasing its activity. Sometimes tetanus affects only the nerves supplying the affected muscle (local tetanus). In others it may enter the blood stream and have a generalized effect. It takes 7-10 days for the symptoms to present after the injury.

Signs and Symptoms:

It is characterized by an increase in muscle tone and spasm of muscles. Initially, the person notices spasm of the masseters (trismus or lockjaw). Soon there is pain and stiffness in the neck, shoulder and back muscles. As the toxin affects more regions, the abdomen and proximal limb muscles become stiff. The spasms of the facial muscles appear as if the individual is grimacing or sneering - risus sardonicus. The contraction of the back muscles may produce an abnormal curvature of the back. In severe cases, the muscles may be thrown into violent spasm with the slightest stimulus threatening the entry of air into the lungs.

The increased activity of the sympathetic system presents as an exaggerated fight or flight response with palpitation, sweating and increased blood pressure.

Complications of tetanus include fractures (due to the violent spasms), pneumonia, muscle rupture, inflammation of veins, decubitus ulcers and muscle death.

Risk factors:

Tetanus can occur in individuals who are not immunized or are partially immunized and in those immunized individuals who have not had the required booster doses. The disease is common in areas where soil is cultivated, in rural areas, in regions with a warmer climate and in summer months. In countries where immunization is not given major importance, tetanus may be seen in newborns.

Tetanus can occur in inadequately cleaned wounds. It may also complicate ulcers, abscesses and gangrene.

Caution and Recommendations to Therapists:

Tetanus is a serious illness that requires hospitalization. However, tetanus is entirely preventable by proper immunization. For adults, the vaccine is given in three doses - the first and second are given 4-8 weeks apart and the third 6-12 months after the second. A booster dose is required every 10 years. Encourage clients to get immunized against tetanus. The therapist should keep a record of her/his own vaccine schedule. Ensure that the clinic has a first aid kit and clean all wounds thoroughly with disinfectant and hydrogen per oxide.

Notes:

Hospitalization is required for tetanus. Tetanus toxoid - antibodies that neutralize the toxin are given immediately to act against free toxins. The course of tetanus lasts for 4-6 weeks. Muscle pain and spasms can last for many months.

Thoracic outlet syndrome

Cardiovascular, Musculoskeletal, Nervous systems

It includes conditions that produce symptoms of pressure on structures that exit from the thorax .

Cause:

This syndrome is caused by entrapment or pressure on structures like nerve

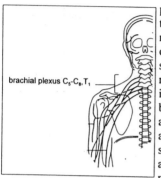

brachial plexus C₅-C₈,T₁

plexuses, arteries and veins, that pass through the thoracic outlet to enter the limbs. Cervical ribs, misaligned ribs, spasm of neck muscles (scalenes) or other muscles like pectoralis minor lying close to the structures passing through the thoracic outlet can result in this syndrome. Scalene Anterior Syndrome, is a term given to conditions that put pressure on the brachial plexus as it passes between the scalene anterior and medius. This may occur due to scaring and adhesions after whiplash injury. Pectoralis syndrome is caused by pressure on the brachial plexus and blood vessels as they pass between the pectoralis minor and coracoid process of the scapula. Costoclavicular syndrome is a term given to conditions that put pressure on the nerves and vessels as they pass between the clavicle and the first rib.

Signs and Symptoms:

Edema or heaviness of the arms, numbness, tingling or weakness of the upperlimb are some of the symptoms.

Risk Factors:

It could be familial if a cervical rib is present in other members of the family. Kyphosis and bad posture may also predispose this condition. Pressure in the armpit as in the use of crutches can also damage the nerves going to the limb. Whiplash injury or similar trauma that produces spasm of the neck muscles are other predisposing factors.

Caution and Recommendations to Therapists:

Assess the range of motion of neck and upper limbs. The pulse may weaken and symptoms may be precipitated or reduced on changing the position of the limb. This indicates the presence of this syndrome.

Massage helps reduce stress, relax muscles and thereby relieve symptoms of this syndrome especially if the cause is spasm of muscles. Position the client as comfortably as possible, using supporting pillows and towels if postural defects are present. Keep the upper limb elevated above the level of the heart, with pillows throughout the treatment if edema is present.

Initially with the client supine, massage the chest, shoulder and neck using broad strokes of effleurage and petrissage. Then concentrate on the muscles of the neck and shoulder, passively moving the neck through the full range of movement. Massage the sternocleidomastoid, trapezius, levator scapulae, pectoralis major and minor and scalene muscles, using special techniques for trigger points and for releasing adhesions. Massage all these muscles from origin to insertion. Use lymphatic drainage techniques on the limb to reduce edema. Deep moist heat can be used to reduce pain and to soften the connective tissue. Fascial stretches,

272

muscle stripping, and exercises are other techniques used. Finish treatment with a whole body relaxing massage.

Encourage client to sleep in a supine position with just one soft pillow under the head.

Inital treatment schedules of twice a week for three weeks have been recommended.

Notes: _____

Tinea versicolor

Integumentary system

A fungal infection of the skin.

Cause:

A fungi malassezia furfur causes this condition.

Signs and Symptoms:

The fungus commonly affects the back and upper chest with lesions that appear scaly and multicolored - from yellow, pink to brown. The patches appear lighter in color as compared to the normal skin as the fungi does not allow the affected area of skin to tan. The client may not take notice of the lesions as they are painless. Often treatment is sought only for cosmetic reasons (see Appendix I figure 14).

Risk factors:

It is more common in those with lowered immunity or diabetes.

Caution and Recommendations to Therapists:

Do not massage clients with lesions. Boil and steam press bedding, towels and clothes if contact has been made. Advice client to get treated.

Notes: _____
Topical antifungal creams have to be used for cure.

Tonsillitis

An inflammation of the tonsils.

Cause:

The inflammation is due to a bacterial infection commonly produced by Beta haemolytic streptococci. The disease spreads by direct contact with respiratory secretions or saliva. The incubation period is 1-3 days. Rarely, it may also be caused by a virus or other bacteria.

Signs and Symptoms:

The person presents with sore throat, difficulty in swallowing, fever and painful

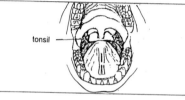

lymph node enlargement. Joint and muscle pain, headache and chills are other symptoms. The symptoms last for 3-7 days. In chronic tonsillitis there is recurrent sore throat with a pustular discharge from the tonsils. Chronic tonsillitis can lead to an abscess formation.

Risk factors:

It is more common in children between the ages of 5-10.

Caution and Recommendations to Therapists:

Encourage client to complete the full course of the prescribed antibiotic treatment which should be for 10-14 days. Increased fluid intake, warm salt water gargling are other forms of treatment used. Do not massage until two days after start of treatment with antibiotics. A therapist with tonsillitis should be excluded from work for at least two days after the start of antibiotic treatment. This is to avoid spreading the infection to clients and others in the work place.

Notes:

The tonsils is a rounded mass of lymphoid tissue located in the pharynx. It is one of the lymphatic organs.

Tooth Decay (Dental caries) Gastrointestinal system

A slow disintegration of the surface of the tooth.

Cause:

The formation of plaques/coating on the surface of the teeth by dead cells, food, bacteria etc. alter the acidity of the environment around the tooth. This results in the demineralisation and disintegration of the tooth.

Signs and Symptoms:

It starts as a blackening of the tooth. If left untreated the tooth is corroded further with resultant tingling and pain. It may be super-infected and become a tooth abscess.

Risk factors:

Unhealthy hygiene of the mouth predisposes to this condition.

Caution and Recommendations to Therapists:

Pain may be referred to other areas of the face depending on the tooth affected. Hydrotherapy may help reduce pain and swelling. If there is an infection, the lymph nodes in the neck may be enlarged. Avoid massaging over enlarged lymph nodes.

Notes:

For tooth extraction, usually the trigeminal nerve is anaesthetized.

Torticollis (Wry-neck) Musculoskeletal system

A malposition of the head and neck due to the shortening of the muscles of the neck such as sternocleidomastoids.

Cause:

It may be congenital or acquired. The congenital form is due to fibrosis or shortening of one of the sternocleidomastoid muscle. It may be due to malpositioning of the fetus inside the uterus, or injury to the neck muscles by forceps delivery. The acquired form, which is rare, could be due to spasm of the muscle on exposure to cold or compression of the nerve supplying the muscle. Whiplash injury can result in injury to and inflammation of the muscle. Healing by fibrosis can cause shortening of the muscle and lead to wry neck.

Signs and Symptoms:

There is shortening of the sternocleidomastoid or hardening of other muscles such as the scalenes, trapezius and splenius. The head is fixed in a bent position with the face tilted. Usually the muscle feels hard but there is no pain. There is scoliosis in the cervical region. In the congenital form there may be associated deformity of the face with the eye and mouth on the affected side drawn down. The nose may be deviated. (The changes in the face disappear once the position of the head is corrected). Pain may be present due to the development of trigger points in the sternocleidomastoid muscle. This pain may be referred to other areas like the ear, cheek and sternum. Autonomic symptoms like watering of the eye, dizziness, ringing in the ear may be present.

Risk factors:

The congenital form is more common in girls. Occupations that require prolonged tilting of the head can predispose to this condition.

Caution and Recommendations to Therapists:

The aim is to relax the neck, stretch the contracted muscle, improve the range of motion and release trigger points. Massage in the seated position may be best for these clients. Lying on the side or supine positions are also well tolerated. Deep moist heat can be used to reduce spasm and soften the connective tissue. Use firm but light strokes with the tips of the fingers. The strokes should be directed along the length of the muscle. Fascial stretching techniques can be used for the contracted muscles. Passive movements of the head with the head over the edge of the table, but well supported with hands help stretch the muscle. The head and shoulder areas should be thoroughly massaged. Care should be taken to avoid pressure over the carotid artery that lies superficially in the neck. In people with narrowed arteries or with inadequate blood flow to the brain, manipulation of the neck may produce dizziness. Avoid turning the head to one side in these individuals people.

Work in close conjunction with the physiotherapist. Encourage client to do remedial exercises to stretch the sternocleidomastoid and scalene muscles.

Initially, massage should be scheduled twice a week for a month, and the frequency altered according to improvement.

Notes: ─────────────────────────────

Toxemia of Pregnancy (Eclampsia, Preeclampsia, Pregnancy - induced Hypertension)

Reproductive system

A condition where there is increased blood pressure, protein loss in the urine and severe edema produced usually after twenty weeks of pregnancy.

Cause:

The cause is not known. It has been thought to be due to the changes in the responsiveness of the blood vessels to circulating hormones. Prostaglandins have been implicated.

Signs and Symptoms:

In a person with this condition, the systolic blood pressure is more than 140 millimeters of Mercury (mmHg) or has increased by 30mmHg or more as compared to previous levels, and the diastolic pressure is above 90 mmHg or has increased by 15mmHg or more than levels before 20th week of pregnancy. There is a gain in weight of more than 3lb per week indicating retention of fluid and edema.The person also passes less than 400 ml. of urine a day (normal about 1000ml). Other associated general symptoms include headache, irritability, heartburn and blurring of vision. The growth of the fetus is also retarded. In the more severe condition - eclampsia, the person has convulsions, with premature labor or still birth. The liver failure may occur in the mother.

Risk factors:

It is more common in pregnant adolescents or those over the age of 35. The incidence is higher in the southeastern parts of the United states.

Caution and Recommendations to Therapists:

Refer pregnant clients to Obstetrician if a sudden increase in weight, or edema is noted. Discourage all pregnant clients from smoking or drinking alcohol. Consult Obstetrician before massaging a client with preeclampsia.

Massage with its psychological relaxing effects can be therapeutic. The effect of massage on the autonomic nervous system can help lower the elevated blood pressure. The client may be massaged seated or turned to the left side. A gentle, relaxing massage of shorter duration is recommended. Do not try to reduce the edema as the underlying cause of edema in this case is due to kidney and liver and not improper drainage of interstitial fluid.

Notes:

The condition is serious because of the complications such as kidney failure, liver failure and persistent hypertension. It is treated with careful monitoring, bed rest, sedatives, anti-convulsants and anti-hypertensives. Due to the threat to the mother, some advocate early induction of labor. Early diagnosis and prompt treatment is required.

The blood pressure in a normal pregnancy decreases during the first trimester being at its lowest during the second trimester.

Transient Ischemic Attack (TIA)

A sudden onset of neurological abnormalities that lasts for less than 24 hours and clears soon after.

Cause:

It is caused by temporary clogging of arterial branches in the brain by small emboli released from thrombi or spasms of arteries that lasts for a short duration.

Signs and Symptoms:

The symptoms are the same as for stroke except that it lasts from a few hours to a day and the person is completely normal again. The symptoms include, speech abnormality, loss of vision, weakness of one side of the body, gait abnormalities, dizziness etc. The symptoms depend on the site of the brain affected.

Risk factors:

There is a higher incidence over the age of 50. It is more common in Afro-Americans and in men.

Caution and Recommendations to Therapists:

See under Stroke. These clients are prone to bleeding if on anticoagulant therapy. Avoid using excessive pressure, as bleeding may occur under the skin.

Notes: _____

A high risk of stroke is present in individuals with TIA. These clients are treated with aspirin and anticoagulants.

Trigeminal neuralgia (Tic douloureux)

A painful condition produced by irritation of the trigeminal nerve (5th cranial nerve).

Cause:

The cause is not known. It may be a reflex phenomena at the sensory nerve level or at the level of the brain. It may also be due to pressure on or reduced blood supply to the nerve.

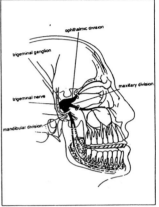

Signs and Symptoms:

It is characterized by excruciating, intermittent pain confined to one or both sides along the distribution of the trigeminal nerve - ie. on the face. The pain may be triggered by any touch or movement such as chewing, eating, swallowing, shaving etc. In some people even a draft of air, exposure to heat or cold may trigger an attack. Trigger zones may be at the tip of the nose, cheeks or gums. The pain may be of burning or jabbing type lasting for a few minutes. There may be a dull ache in the region between attacks. Many people are symptom-free between attacks.

Risk factors:

Scarring, pressure on the 5th cranial nerve can predispose to this. It is more common over the age of 40 with a higher incidence in women than men. It may occur in individuals with multiple sclerosis or shingles.

Caution and Recommendations to Therapists:

Get a good history of the signs and symptoms and treatment and get clearance from a physician. Make a note of possible triggers to an attack. The individual may not allow you to touch the side of face where attacks occur. In such cases, avoid the local area and do a general relaxation massage.

If the client finds massage beneficial, initially use effleurage and friction over the skull with the client in a seated position. Use effleurage for about two minutes then stroke gently and continuously starting from the middle of the face towards the temple and periphery. Start in the least sensitive area and move towards sensitive areas. Do not overwork specific areas as it may irritate the nerve and cause more pain. Do not repeat the strokes more than thrice in one area.The duration of the massage should be for 10 minutes with almost half the time spent on the skull. Schedule a total of 10-15 treatments at a frequency of one treatment every day or every other day.

Notes: _____

Tuberculosis (Phthisis, Consumption, TB)

Respiratory, Gastrointestinal, Renal, Nervous, Musculoskeletal, Lymphatic systems

An acute or chronic bacterial infection that primarily affects the lungs. It may affect any system in the body.

Cause:

The infection is caused by the bacteria Mycobacterium tuberculosis. The bacteria is transmitted by airborne droplets that are produced by infected individuals when they cough, sneeze or talk. The droplets can remain suspended in the air or be transported over long distances. It may also be spread by ingestion eg. milk from a tuberculous cow - leading to tuberculosis of the gastrointestinal tract. The incubation period is 4-12 weeks. The bacteria causes a reaction in the lungs when they are inhaled. The macrophages ward off the infection by forming fibrous tubercles around the infected site which may later become calcified. Here the bacteria can lie dormant over years and get reactivated when the individuals are susceptible. The tissue reaction may progress to formation of cavities and fibrosis in the lungs.

> **To ponder....**
>
> * About one-third of the world's population - 1.7 billion people are infected with TB
>
> * About eight million people develop active TB each year
>
> * About three million people die from this disease each year

Signs and Symptoms:

Initially, the individual is asymptomatic. Respiratory tuberculosis presents as chronic cough and blood in sputum. Low grade fever, weight loss and fatigue are other general symptoms.

Risk factors:

People living in crowded, poorly ventilated buildings and those malnourished are at higher risk. Uncontrolled diabetes, AIDS, Hodgkin's disease, silicosis, individuals on corticosteroids/immunosuppressants and substance abusers are prone. It is more common in infants and the elderly.

Caution and Recommendations to Therapists:

In general, tuberculosis is not infectious from 2-4 weeks after start of adequate treatment with antitubercular drugs. Do not massage unless sure that the client is no longer infective. Consult physician regarding infectivity of individuals. Be cautious while treating clients with history of prolonged cough (more than 3 weeks), weight loss, fatigue and low grade fever. Refer such clients to a physician before you treat. Massage therapists should periodically get screened for tuberculosis by skin tests. Keep track of the epidemiology of tuberculosis in your area. If exposed to tuberculosis inadvertently, consult physician immediately and watch for results of skin testing and take preventive treatment. Ensure that the local exhaust and general ventilation of the clinic is functioning properly.

Notes:

Tuberculin Skin testing or Mantoux test is done to screen individuals. A positive test only indicates that the person has been exposed to tuberculosis. It does not indicate that the individual is infectious.

Not all TB patients are infectious ie. able to spread the disease. Only 10% of individuals progress to active disease. Individuals are infectious only when the disease is active. The majority of individuals enter a latent phase from which there is a lifelong risk of reactivation. If a therapist has active tuberculosis, work should not be resumed unless cleared by physician ie. until three consecutive sputum smears are negative for tuberculous bacilli and clinical improvement is seen. TB is treated with multiple drugs for at least 6-9 months.

Tuberculosis - bone (Pott's disease)

Musculoskeletal system

Tuberculous infection of bone, usually the spine.

Cause:

It is caused by an infection of the spine by Mycobacterium tuberculosis. The infection is usually spread from another part of the body such as the lungs or lymph nodes.

Signs and Symptoms:

There is bone destruction and abscess formation. The lower thoracic vertebrae are most frequently affected. The vertebrae collapse under the weight of the body with deformity of the spine. The client feels pain at the site of the infection. Referred pain may be felt along the dermatome if there is pressure on the roots of the nerve.

The spasm of the back muscles immobilize the affected spine and produce rigidity in the area. The gait and posture is altered in order to support the affected vertebrae. Angular deformities of the spine can be seen. Complications include abscess formation, compression of nerves and spinal cord by the collapsed vertebrae and spread to other areas.

Risk factors:

Tuberculosis is more common in people of poor hygiene, living in overcrowded homes. (See Tuberculosis - lung). Bone TB is seen more frequently in children.

Caution and Recommendations to Therapists:

Acute cases are treated by immobilization and anti-tuberculous drugs. Consult physician and ensure that the client is not infective. Encourage client to take the full course of treatment. If the client is not infectious, massage may be given to the unaffected areas.

Notes: _____

Typhoid fever (Enteric fever)   Gastrointestinal system

An acute bacterial infection that affects many systems.

Cause:

It is usually caused by the bacteria Salmonella typhi. Other species Salmonella paratyphi A, paratyphi B may also cause the disease. Most often it spreads from a carrier who may harbor the bacteria for over 50 years. Contamination of water or food by a human carrier is the most common form of spread of disease. Carriers may harbor the virus in their gall bladder from where it enters the intestines through the bile and is excreted in the feces.

The organism on being ingested enter the small intestines. They can multiply inside macrophages and monocytes that engulf them. Soon the organism enters the gall bladder and other areas. The incubation period is variable and depends on the immunity of the host and the number of organisms ingested and may extend from 3-60 days.

Signs and Symptoms:

It presents as prolonged high fever associated with headache, apathy and chills. If untreated the fever may last for 4-8 weeks. Ulcers in the intestine may cause indigestion, bleeding and sometimes perforation. The chances of perforation is highest in the third or fourth week after symptoms. There may be tenderness and swelling of the liver and spleen. Often abdominal pain is present. Sometimes, rashes may be seen over the chest and abdomen in the first week of infection. Complications of typhoid can occur in almost all systems.

Risk factors:

Those travelling to endemic areas such as Mexico, Pakistan, India, Chile and Peru are at higher risk. Also, the incidence is higher in individuals with a lowered immunity such as those with AIDS, the elderly etc.

Caution and Recommendations to Therapists:

Ensure that the clients with a history of typhoid are not carriers. In those clients recovering from typhoid it is important to avoid the abdominal area during massage as it takes sometime for the intestinal ulcers to heal, and the swelling of the liver and spleen to subside.

Encourage clients to get vaccinated before travelling to areas that are endemic for typhoid.

Notes: ───

Urinary tract infection

Renal system

An infection of one or more structures of the urinary tract.

Cause:

It is caused by bacteria when the local defenses in the bladder are broken down.

Signs and Symptoms:

Frequency of urination, burning sensation on passing urine are the common symptoms. The urine may be blood stained and cloudy. Fever, low back pain and tenderness over the suprapubic area are other symptoms.

Risk factors:

It is more common in women due to the shortness of the urethra. Any kind of obstruction in the urinary tract predisposes to this infection. Catheterization, pregnancy, loss of bladder control as in spinal cord injuries, renal stones, birth defects of the urinary tract make a person more susceptible to infection.

Caution and Recommendation to Therapists:

Encourage client to take the full course of antibiotics and increase the intake of water to at least eight glasses a day. Urinary tract infection does not spread from person to person unless the local defenses of a person is affected. Tailor massage according to individual needs.

Notes: _____

Inflammation of the urethra is known as urethritis. Pyelonephritis denotes infection of the kidney.

Varicose ulcers   Cardiovascular system

Chronic ulcers in the leg.

Cause:

It is seen in individuals with varicose veins. The sluggish flow of blood in the legs makes the skin prone to injury. Healing is also delayed and this results in ulceration.

Signs and Symptoms:

Slow onset of ulcers in the medial aspect of the leg in a person who has varicose veins is typical. There is edema and congestion of blood vessels. The ulcer may follow a mild injury to the leg with varicose veins, which later gets infected. Healing is sluggish due to the poor circulation in the limb. The skin around the ulcer may be hardened, edematous and discolored. The hardening is due to slow healing by fibrosis which further compromises the blood flow to the area. If there is superinfection the client will have fever, and signs of inflammation - redness, heat, swelling and pain. There may be pus discharge from the ulcer and the ulcer may appear yellow or white (see Appendix I figure 15).

Risk factors:

See Varicose veins.

Caution and Recommendations to Therapists:

These clients are prone for thrombosis. After clearance from the physician, the therapist should aim to reduce edema and prevent venous and lymphatic stasis. The client should be massaged with the leg raised above the level of the heart. To reduce edema and congestion, deep and slow effleurage and kneading movements should be used starting from the thigh and continuing down the limb. To soften the hardening around the ulcer and to improve circulation, deep friction around the ulcer should be employed.

Notes: _____

Varicose veins

Abnormally dilated and tortuous veins of the lower limbs or other areas. In the esophagus, veins are dilated when the blood is shunted from the abdomen to the thorax through alternative routes when the architecture of the liver is distorted as in cirrhosis.

Cause:

The veins in the limbs in general are of two types - superficial and deep. The superficial veins (the long and short saphenous veins in the lower legs) drain blood from the skin and subcutaneous areas which in turn flow into the deeper veins via communicating veins. Valves, as well as the pumping action of the surrounding skeletal muscles, prevent back flow. In clients with varicose veins, prolonged dilatation and stretching of the vessel wall make the valves incompetent and result in backflow and stagnation of blood in the veins of the lower limbs.

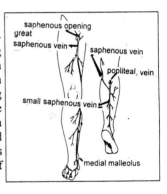

Varicose veins may be primary or secondary. When the varicosity is due to the superficial veins the cause is said to be primary. Secondary varicose veins result from defects in the deep veins. The latter may be due to infection of the veins - thrombophlebitis.

Varicosities can also occur in other areas like the esophagus, rectum. (See Esophageal varices and Hemorrhoids)

Signs and Symptoms:

The client complains of pain or ache in the lower legs, especially on using them.

They may also complain of progressive heaviness of the leg on prolonged standing. Some edema may be present.

Tortuous veins may be visible. In those clients with prolonged varicose veins, ulcers may be seen. Also, superficial injuries take a longer time to heal in these clients. (See Appendix I figure 15)

Risk Factors:

Varicose veins are more common in clients whose occupation requires prolonged standing. The hormones, estrogen and progesterone relax the smooth muscles of the veins thus making women more prone for venous insufficiency. The risk is even higher during pregnancy. Varicose veins may also be familial as it has been shown that the number and competency of the valves in the veins differs from person to person. Obesity also predisposes to varicose veins.

Caution and Recommendations to Therapists:

In those with MILD varicosity, light, local massage helps move blood and lymph towards the heart. If possible keep the leg elevated for 15 to 30 minutes before massage and throughout the treatment period to use the effects of gravity on venous drainage. The aim is to help blood flow in the collateral circulation. Use strokes such as effleurage, kneading, squeezing and picking up. Massage the proximal areas before moving to the distal areas. This helps decongest the proximal blood vessels that eventually drain blood from the distal vessels. If the short saphenous vein is affected, massage first the thigh then the anterior tibial group and finally the calf. Avoid massage directly over the dilated vein. Gentle passive movements of the joints are also helpful. If the client is on supporting bandages or stocking, remove the bandage after the positioning of the client and reapply before the client gets off the table.

DO NOT MASSAGE OVER SEVERE VARICOSITIES. In those clients with twisted and hard veins, with ulceration and edema, local massage is contraindicated as prolonged stasis in the veins tend to promote thrombi formation. Massage can dislodge the thrombus if present. The emboli thus formed can in turn block arteries in the lungs, heart or brain and result in pulmonary edema, myocardial infarction, or stroke respectively. A simple test (Homan's sign) to eliminate the possibility of thrombosis in the deep vein is to dorsiflex the foot with the knee extended. If the client complains of pain in the calf it may indicate presence of deep vein thrombus.

Another complication of severe varicose veins is rupture of the weak walls with even the slightest of injuries. If such an emergency occurs call a physician. Apply firm pressure pads above and below the injury with the client lying with the leg well raised.

Always consult the attending physician if the varicosity is chronic.

Advice client to keep leg elevated above heart level whenever possible. For those clients who have had surgery, massage helps relieve the general fatigue in the legs. Use deep transverse friction strokes over the incision scars to prevent adhesions.

Notes: ──

Varicose veins are treated with elastic bandages or stockings and exercise programs, in mild cases. In chronic or severe cases surgery is done where the vein may be stripped (removed), ligated (tied off) or destroyed with a sclerosing agent.

═══

Venous thrombosis Cardiovascular system

Presence of thrombus in a vein. (A thrombus is a blood clot attached to the walls of a blood vessel.)

Cause:

Clotting is a natural phenomenon which prevents loss of blood, by clogging abnormal or potential openings in the vessel wall. Factors that promote clotting in the blood vessel such as stagnation of blood, injury to the vessel wall and alteration in the coaguability of blood promote thrombus formation.

Venous thrombosis can form in superficial or deep veins and is more common in the veins of the lower limbs. The major complication of thrombosis is the formation of emboli and resultant pulmonary edema, myocardial infarction or stroke.

Signs and Symptoms:

Since a thrombus is accompanied by inflammation in the vessel wall - thrombo-phlebitis, the client can present with pain, swelling, and muscle tenderness in and around the local area. The arterial pulse in the leg may be reduced or absent and the leg may appear pale. Fever and general malaise may also be present. In individuals with deep vein thrombosis, pain in the calf is felt if the ankle is dorsiflexed with the knee extended (Homan's sign).

Risk factors:

Prolonged bed rest and immobilization, absence of blood factors which prevent clotting, or increased levels of factors like fibrinogen that promote clotting predispose to the formation of venous thrombosis. Increased levels of clotting factors are seen in those using oral contraceptives as well as during, and soon after pregnancy. Infections, trauma, surgery and catheterization also promote thrombi formation.

Caution and Recommendations to Therapists:

Local massage is contraindicated in venous thrombosis. Apart from increasing the pain and inflammation, the thrombus can be dislodged resulting in major complications including death.

In a client under treatment for venous thrombosis, massage should be done only in consultation with the physician. Since treatment for thrombosis includes drugs which inhibit clotting, such clients have bleeding tendencies and deep massage can result in small bleeds (petechiae, ecchymosis) under the skin. See Appendix I figure 10.

Notes: ───

Deep vein thrombosis is treated with strict bed rest and prolonged anticoagulant therapy.

Vitiligo

Integumentary system

White irregular patches on the skin.

Cause:

The cause is unknown. But there is loss of pigment cells in the area.

Signs and Symptoms:

Hypopigmented patches are seen on the skin. The patches may be symmetrical and bilateral, and are more common around the eyes, mouth, and body folds. There may not be any inflammation.

Risk factors:

The incidence is higher between 10 and 30 years of age. There may be a family history. It may be associated with other diseases like thyroid disease, Addison's disease, diabetes mellitus etc. Stress, severe sunburn, surgery or pregnancy may precipitate vitiligo.

Caution and Recommendations to Therapists:

Infection by tinea versicolor (which is infectious) should be ruled out. Apart from the cosmetic effects, vitiligo is a harmless condition. A high degree of sensitivity to the emotional needs of the client is required in the part of the therapist.

Notes: _____

Techniques to increase pigmentation are employed to treat this condition. Creams and exposure to sunlight/ultraviolet light are used.

Vulvitis

An inflammation of the female external genitalia - vulva.

Cause:

It is commonly caused by yeast (candida albicans) infection. It may also be transmitted sexually in which case it may be of viral origin. Other causes may be a reaction to chemicals such as laundry products, soaps, sprays etc. In older women, symptoms may be due to atrophy of the tissue with age.

Signs and Symptoms:

Severe itching is the commonest symptom.

Risk factors:

It is common in those with diabetes mellitus.

Caution and Recommendations to Therapists:

Have clients wear underclothes during treatment.

Notes: _____

The vulva includes the structures - labia majora, labia minora, mons pubis, clitoris and adjacent areas.

Vulvitis is treated according to the cause. General measures include keeping the area dry and clean, and decrease itching by application of cortisol cream.

Warts (Condylomata acuminata, Veruca vulgaris)

A viral infection commonly affecting the genital area producing a fleshy growth.

Cause:

Warts are caused by the human papilloma virus. Anogenital warts are caused by a different strain of virus as compared to the strain causing warts in other areas. The incubation period is 2-3 months. The papilloma virus is transmitted by sexual or intimate contact with an affected individual. However, not all people who have come in contact get the disease.

Signs and Symptoms:

Warts are painless, fleshy, multiple growths seen on the surface of skin. In the dry skin, they appear as pink growths of different consistency, sizes and shapes - soft, cauliflower like, or flat and granular, or small, pointed and firm. In males, warts occur more commonly on the penis or in the anal area. In females, they may appear in the external genitalia or anal region.(see Appendix I figure 16)

Risk factors:

Direct contact with an infected person puts one at risk. Smoking, immuno suppression, other sexually transmitted diseases and oral contraceptives increase the risk of contracting the disease. As well, these factors place an infected person at a higher risk for malignant changes.

Caution and Recommendations to Therapists:

Observe strict hygienic procedures while massaging all clients. Avoid massaging individuals with warts and advice medical treatment as it is a precancerous condition.

Notes:

Whiplash (Acceleration Deceleration injury)

Musculoskeletal system

A condition produced by damage to muscles, ligaments, inter vertebral disks and nerve tissues of the cervical region by sudden hyperextension and/or flexion of neck.

Cause:

The commonest cause is automobile accidents - especially the type where an immobile car is struck from behind. The inertia of the head in relation to the body results in hyperextension of the neck. Whiplash can also result from contact sports such as football, or high velocity sports such as skiing. There may be micro or complete tearing of the sternocleidomastoid muscle, longus coli muscle and the anterior longitudinal ligament of the vertebral column. The cervical intervertebral disk may be prolapsed or torn away from the vertebral body.

Signs and Symptoms:

Symptoms start immediately in severe injury. In mild cases, the symptoms may start after 12-24 hours. There is pain in the anterior and posterior regions of the neck. The cervical muscles may be rigid to touch due to the spasm. There is pain, swelling, stiffness, spasm and soreness of the sternocleidomastoid. The skin may be warm and red indicating signs of inflammation.

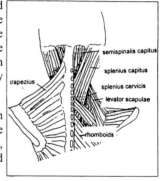

Different groups of muscles are affected depending on the type of injury. In an extension injury, the sternocleidomastoid, scalenes, infrahyoid, suprahyoid, levator scapulae, longus coli, suboccipitals and rhomboids are likely to be injured.

In a flexion type of injury, the trapezius, splenius capitus, semispinalis capitus - ie. muscles behind the neck are likely to be injured.

An injury from the side is likely to affect the sternocleidomastoid, suboccipitals, levator scapulae, splenius capitus, splenius cervicis. Muscles of the upper and lower limbs may be injured in association with those of the neck. The pectoralis major and minor may be injured by the seatbelt.

Disturbances of the vestibular apparatus of the inner ear may result in dizziness, nausea and vomiting, headache and gait disturbances. Disturbance of the cochlea of the inner ear may result in tinnitus (ringing in the ear). Injury to the nerves exiting from the cervical region, may produce numbness in the arms.

Whiplash may also present as restlessness, mood changes and insomnia if concussion to the brain has occurred in addition.

Risk factors:

The risk is increased if driving without proper seatbelt and padded headrests.

Caution and Recommendations to Therapists:

Consult physician about the extent of the injury. Assessment should be done very cautiously in the acute phase. Assess the active range of movement of the cervical spine and shoulder girdle. The acute phase is assessed by the physical findings and not by the duration of the symptoms. This phase may last up to 2-3 weeks. The client may be treated seated or lying to the side. Use hot compresses to neck to relieve pain and spasm in acute cases. Cold compresses may be used to reduce edema. If tolerated by the client, passively move the neck within limits of pain to maintain range of motion. Lymphatic drainage techniques may be used in the shoulder and neck regions.

The subacute phase, is when the pain and swelling of the muscle has subsided. There is no tenderness of muscle. However, pain may be referred to the interscapular region, upper limbs, head and shoulders. Thoroughly massage the back and shoulders using broad strokes. There may be tender points in the sternocleidomastoid, suboccipital, multifidis and other neck muscles. The aim of treatment in this phase is to increase the flexibility of the neck. Stretching exercises should be used.

Stretch the sternocleidomastoid by rotation and lateral flexion. Massage the sternocleidomastoid from origin to insertion using gentle friction strokes. For this to be effective, the client should be in a supine position with the therapist sitting at the head. Grasp the sternocleidomastoid between thumb and fingers and roll and massage the muscle between the fingers. Gently stretch the muscle by running the hand from the head toward the sternum with the head held slightly flexed in the opposite direction of the muscle being stretched.

Stretch to the suboccipital muscle can be produced by mild traction to the occiput. The scalenus muscle can be stretched by rotating the head towards the side of muscle to be stretched and laterally flexing away from the side to be stretched. Isometric exercises can be used to strengthen the multifidis. With the client lying prone and head over the table, support head with hand and slowly allow the client to take the weight of the head and maintain the position at different degrees of extension. Do not overstretch as it may damage the delicate facet joints of the vertebra.

In the chronic phase, the healing is complete but the muscles may be shortened by fibrosis with limitation of the range of motion. The posture may be altered with the head thrust forward. Deep,aching pain may be present. Deep moist heat can be used to reduce pain. Passively move joints, taking care not to overstretch. Use friction massage over the sternocleidomastoid and other neck muscles. Vigorous rotation and stretching should be avoided. Remember that in the case of whiplash it is better to undertreat than overtreat.

Initially, treatment scheduled for half hour duration at a frequency of two to three times a week for two weeks is recommended. The frequency may be reduced to one or two times a week for another two weeks and then rescheduled after assessment.

Since law suits may be involved in whiplash injury, keep accurate records of assessment and treatment and do not allow access of any other individual to the records.

Notes: _____

The prognosis of the injury is related to the direction of the initial impact. In general, prognosis is worst for those involved in accidents where the impact was from the rear (symptoms persist up to or beyond a year after accident). It is a little better in impacts from the side (symptoms last for a few months). The best prognosis is for those involved in head on collisions (symptoms last a few weeks). The extent of injury is less in flexion injuries as the movement of the neck is limited by the chin in front and the shoulder in the side. Extension injuries are worse as the backward movement is not limited unless a high head rest is present.

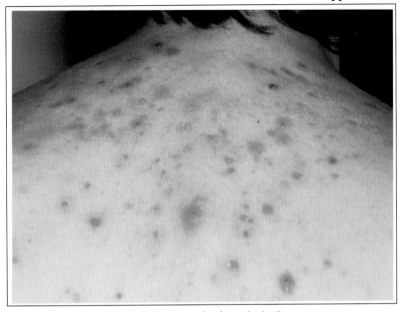

Fig.1 **Acne:** Inflammation of sebaceous glands on the back.

Fig.2 **Athlete's foot:** Fungal infection on the sole of the foot.

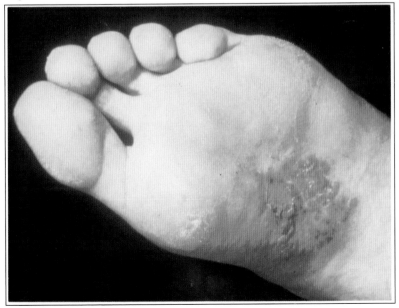

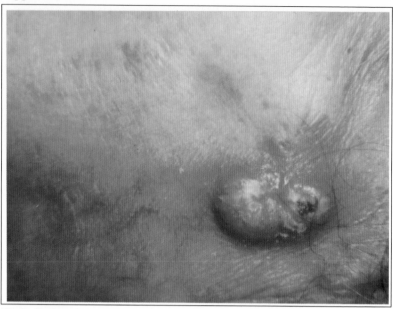

Fig.3 **Carbuncle:** Localised collection of pus with inflammation.

Fig.4 **Gangrene:** Dry and scaly skin with blackened dead tissue.

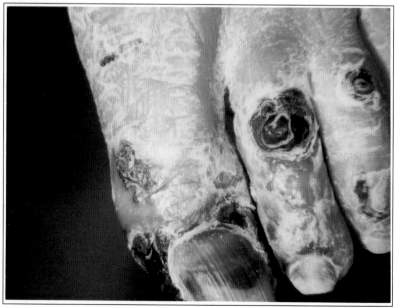

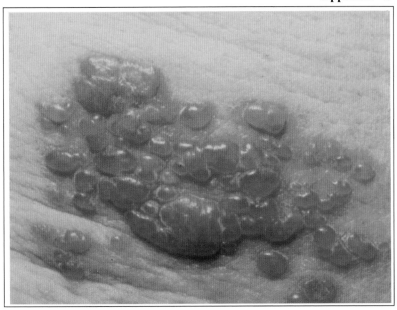

Fig.5 **Herpes Zoster:** Fluid filled crops of vesicles along the distribution of a sensory nerve.

Fig.6 **Impetigo Contagiosa:** Pustular vesicles covered by honey-colored crusts.

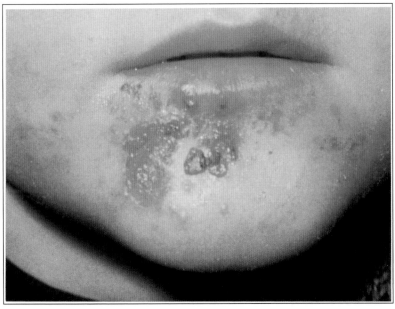

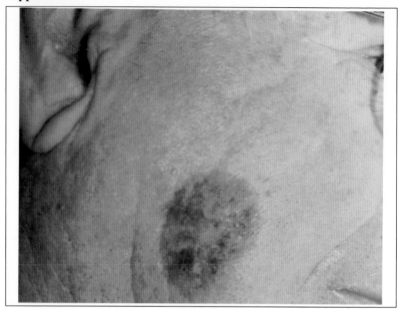

Fig.7 **Malignant Melanoma:** A pigmented lesion with an irregular border, on the face.

Fig.8 **Molluscum Contagiosum:** Pearl like, dimpled crops of lesions.

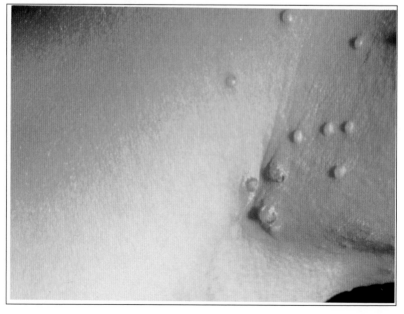

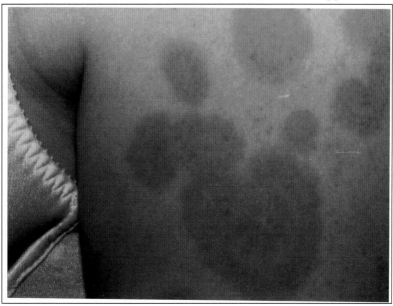

Fig.9 **Psoriasis:** Well defined red patches with thick, silvery, adherent scales.

Fig.10 **Purpura:** Tiny purpulish spots indicating bleeding under the skin. Seen in bleeding disorders, platelet deficiency and collagen disorders.

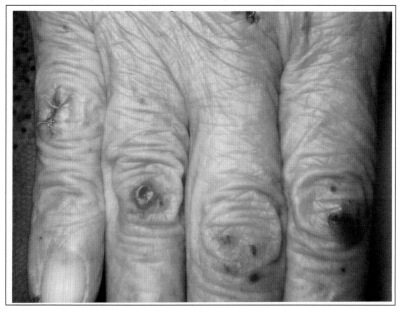

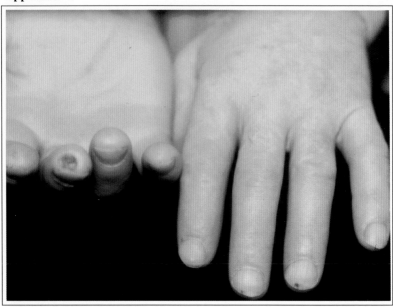

Fig.11 **Scleroderma:** Pale and edematous skin with absence of wrinkles.

Fig.12 **Systemic Lupus Erythematosus:** Typical butterfly rash on the face.

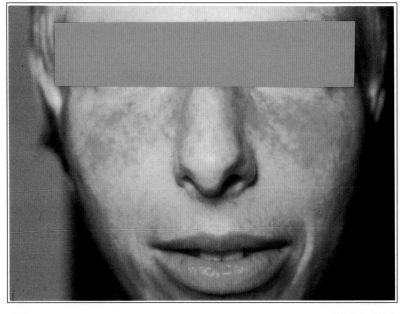

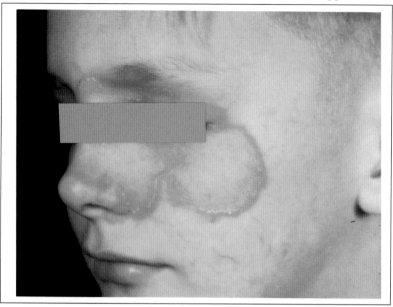

Fig.13 **Tinea Corporis:** Raised and red outline of the lesion with clearing in the central region.

Fig.14 **Tinea Versicolor:** Pale tan patches on the upper trunk.

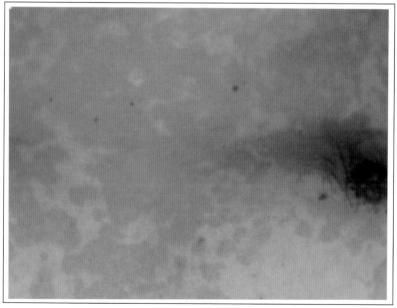

Appendix - I

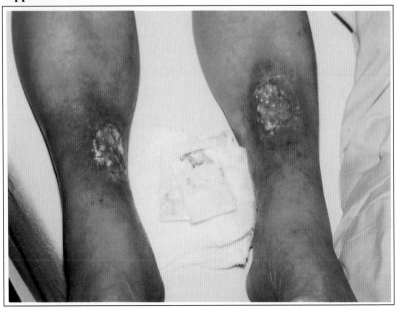

Fig.15 **Ulcers:** A result of chronic stagnation of venous blood eg. a complication of varicose veins.

Fig.16 **Warts:** Irregular and branched crops of lesions on the face.

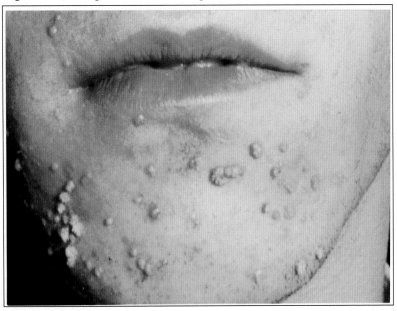

Strategies for Infection Prevention and Safe Practice

Information about clients:

* Always ensure confidentiality of information, especially health related, imparted by the client.

* Maintain a written record of every client seen by you and take a detailed history of past and present illness.

* Obtain the address for a contact person and treating Physician for every client treated.

Spread of infection:

* Remember that blood, and other secretions/excretions of the body are potentially infectious material.

* Remember that disease can be transmitted by:

　　a) contact: *direct* - person to person such as kissing, touching, sexual intercourse, fecal and oral contact and *indirect* - via equipment, bedding, handkerchiefs, linen etc.

　　b) droplet mechanisms such as sneezing, coughing, talking, singing etc. and airborne mechanisms: Light viruses and bacteria can be carried by dust particles and small droplets in air currents.

　　c) vehicle: substances that maintain the life of the agent until it is ingested or inoculated into the susceptible host eg. water, blood, serum, food, feces.

　　d) vector: insects etc. that transmit agents by biting the susceptible host or by depositing the agent on skin or food eg. mosquito, ticks, flies, rats.

* Avoid eating, drinking, smoking and applying lip balm or contact lenses in the clinic area.

* Do not allow pets in area (except seeing eye dogs) as they may be carriers of vectors. Also, some clients may be allergic to hair/fur.

* Request clients to take a shower before coming in for massage.

* Do not treat clients who are immunocompromised - such as clients with AIDS,

immunosuppressed on long-term corticosteroid treatment or on chemotherapy if you have any infection even if mild, as it can lead to serious or fatal infection in such susceptible individuals.

Vaccination and skin tests:

* Get vaccinated. Encourage clients to get vaccinated. Vaccines are available against Hepatitis B virus, influenza, measles, mumps, rubella, poliomyelitis, diphtheria, tetanus among others.

* Periodically get a skin test done for tuberculosis (TB). The frequency of testing varies from area to area according to the incidence of TB and risk assessment.

Care of hands:

* Keep finger nails short and avoid wearing rings, bracelets, or other jewellery that might come in contact with clients while massaging.

* Wash hands with hot water and soap before and after treating clients. Hand washing is the easiest and most effective form of infection control. Vigorous mechanical friction while hand washing is an important component. Do not forget to scrub the nail beds and webs between the fingers and thumb.

* Use plain or antimicrobial soap. If using bar soap, use small bars that can be changed frequently and soap racks that promote drainage. Automatic dispensers are better still.

* Use disposable paper towels rather than cloth for hand drying. If feasible, use hot air.

* Put up a notice above sink and toilet to remind clients to wash hands after using the wash room.

* Wear vinyl or latex gloves if there is a potential chance of touching body fluids or secretions and remove gloves immediately after use and dispose in a leakproof plastic bag. *Wash hands immediately after removing gloves.* Do not reuse gloves.

* If you have been inadvertently exposed to infectious agents, vigorously scrub the site with disinfectant solution such as 10% povidone iodine and wash with

running tap water.

Care of clinic:

* Wash linen - sheets, towels etc. in washer using detergent and hot water. Add one cup of household bleach to each load of laundry. Dry using the hot cycle.

* Ensure that the local exhaust and general ventilation is working adequately in the clinic. The ventilation should be regularly monitored.

* Disinfect clinic regularly including door knobs, and keep written record of the frequency of disinfecting. 70-90% ethyl or isopropyl alcohol is adequate. Follow the product label for dilution while using germicidal detergent solutions.

* Use towels to cover ice/hot packs or other objects that are reused and come in direct contact with clients.

* Periodically clean ice/ice machines.

* Carpets are harder to clean than other floors, consider alternate floor style in massage area.

* A `firstaid kit' should be maintained in the clinic and the contents checked and replenished regularly.

Client education:

* Keep brochures, articles on health, health magazines and pamphlets at vantage points for use by clients while waiting in the clinic.

Self education:

* Be well informed about infectious diseases so that you can recognize them in your client and avoid further harm to the client, yourself or others visiting the clinic.

* Keep reference books, medical dictionary and other resource materials in the clinic for easy and ready reference about rare disorders.

* Read the health sections of newspapers to be aware of local endemics and epidemics.

* Join local, national and international massage organization and subscribe to journals to be current with progress màde in the field and other health related issues.

Commonly used drugs/therapy and adverse effects

Introduction

Along with their beneficial effects drugs are linked with the risk of adverse effects. Aside from the illness/death produced, the adverse effects of drugs complicate diagnosis as they can involve almost all organs and systems of the body. The incidence of adverse effects is increased in the elderly as the number of drugs taken by them at a given time is more than others. Over the counter drugs - nonprescription drugs are common causes of side effects as, frequently, the right dosage is not taken.

In general, the most frequent type of adverse effect is from an exaggeration of the actual, required action of the drug. Other side effects are due to the toxic effect of the drug on organs and systems unrelated to the predicted action. These may be direct toxic effects on tissues, triggering of abnormal immune responses by the body or changes in the metabolic processes of the body especially in those people with genetic enzyme defects.

The exaggeration of the actual action may be due to increased levels of the drug at the site of action. This risk is increased if the drug is not metabolized at the expected rate - as in liver dysfunction, or excreted at a slower rate as in kidney disease. Also, other drugs taken simultaneously may interfere with the breakdown and excretion of a drug.

The magnitude of drug-induced disease is large. It has been estimated that 2-5% of patients admitted in hospitals are due to drug induced disease. Ninety percent of the reactions are produced by a small group of widely used drugs as those given below. The description given here deal with some common agents and their common side-effects, to give the massage therapist an overview - though a superficial one. Also, the given examples of drugs is not an exhaustive list.

Antiasthmatics

Although elimination of the causative agent from the environment is the most successful means for treating asthma, drugs are often needed to prevent or reduce the severity of an attack. The mode of action of the drugs used vary. In general, they relax the smooth muscles of the bronchus and reduce the congestion and inflammation. Some drugs prevent the release of histamine and other molecules from mast cells. Since relaxation of the bronchial smooth muscles is brought about by the sympathetic nervous system, the drugs resemble the neurotransmitters released by the sympathetic nerves viz. noradrenaline. The drugs may also be in the form of antagonists to the neurotransmitters released by the parasympathetic nerves viz. acetylcholine as the parasympathetic system has the opposite action of the sympathetic. Steroids help reduce symptoms through their antiinflammatory and other effects. Thus a single or a combination of drugs can be used in asthma. To increase the local effect and reduce the adverse reactions, many of these drugs are taken as inhalations.

examples: Adrenergic stimulants - epinephrine, isoproterenol, isoetharine, rimiterol, hexoprenaline, salbutamol, albuterol, terbutaline, fenoterol; Methyl xanthines - theophylline; Mast cell stabilizing agents - cromolyn sodium, nedocromil sodium; Anticholinergics - atropine, ipratropium bromide

Common side effects:

The side effects resemble that of excessive sympathetic stimulation ie *fight or flight reaction.* One of the common side effects of the adrenergic stimulants is *cardiac arrhythmias.* The methyl xanthines may cause *nervousness, vomiting, anorexia* and *headache.*

Anticoagulants

Anticoagulants are given to those who have a tendency to develop or have developed thrombi in the blood vessels. For example, it is used in those with deep vein thrombosis and heart disease.

examples: heparin, warfarin, urokinase, streptokinase

Common side effects:

The most common side effect is the *tendency to bleed.* Anticoagulants increase the chances of bleeding especially in those who are predisposed - eg. in those with active bleeding, bleeding tendency, uncontrolled hypertension, pregnancy and during/after surgery.

As a therapist, special care should be taken not to use excessive pressure as bleeding may occur under the skin. In some cases, the bleeding can be fatal.

Antidiabetics

Diabetes is treated in many ways. The goal of the treatment is to maintain the glucose levels as close to normal at all times and thereby prevent/ reduce complications. Diabetes can produce complications in almost all systems of the body. Mild diabetes is treated by changes in lifestyle and dietary habits. Diabetes that cannot be controlled conservatively, has to be treated with oral antidiabetic drugs or insulin. Since insulin is a protein and can be digested in the intestines, it has to be given in the form of injections.

examples: sulfonylurea (glyburide, glipizide, tolazamide, acetohexamide), biguanide (metformin), insulin

Common side effects:
Hypoglycemia is the most common side effect. Hypoglycemia may manifest as sweating, palpitation, anxiety, giddiness and coma. The therapist should ensure that all diabetics have their drugs handy when they come for massage. A contact address should also be recorded in case of emergencies. Since prolonged hypoglycemia can produce irreversible brain damage, glucose has to be administered to the diabetic client as soon as possible if they present with symptoms of hypoglycemia. Sometimes giddiness and coma may be due to *hyperglycemia*. This can occur if the dosage and frequency of administration of the antidiabetic agent is wrong.

Other toxic reactions include *skin rash* and *jaundice*. In the case of clients on insulin, sterile abscesses may form at the site of injection. Common sites of injection are the anterior abdominal wall, anterior aspect of the thigh, buttocks, posterior aspect of the arm. Special care should be taken while massaging injection sites as it is important for these areas to be clean. Also, massage over an injection site can speed up the absorption of insulin and cause a sudden drop in glucose levels in the blood. *Insulin allergy* is another adverse effect. Itching, swelling and redness of the injection site may be seen. in those clients who inject insulin at the same site, *lipohypertrophy* (increased fat accumulation) may be seen. *Lipoatrophy* may be seen in injection sites if impure insulin is injected.

Antihistamines

These drugs are given to reduce itching and to control inflammation. They antagonise the secretion and action of histamine which is responsible for the itching, swelling and redness, particularly prominent in allergic conditions.

example: diphenhyrdamine, chlorpheneramine, tripelenamine hydroxyzine, loratadine, astemizole, terfenadine

Common side effects:
One of the common side effects of antihistamines is its *sedatory effects.* They may also cause excessive *dryness of the mouth and nose. Rebound rhinitis* is seen when the antihistamines given for allergic rhinitis is discontinued. Systemically, these drugs can cause *irritability, insomnia* and *hypertension.*

Antihypertensives

The aim of antihypertensive treatment is to prevent the long-term sequelae such as strokes, myocardial infarction etc. Although mild forms of hypertension can be controlled by alteration of life style and dietary habits, moderate to severe forms require treatment with drugs that need to be taken over a long period.

In general, antihypertensive drugs reduce the blood pressure by relaxing the smooth muscles of blood vessels. This is done by reducing the activity of the sympathetic nervous system - by affecting the areas in the brain regulating the system or by giving drugs that reduce the availability of the neurotransmitters secreted by the sympathetic nervous system at its nerve endings. Calcium channel blockers are other mechanisms by which the smooth muscle of blood vessels can be relaxed. Diuretics may also be given to reduce blood pressure. This acts by reducing the blood volume and the plasma level of sodium. Some drugs act by inhibiting hormones that normally tend to increase blood pressure. All of the above have the potential to produce adverse effects that are due to excessive sympathetic suppression.

examples: atenolol, betaxolol, metoprolol, nadolol, timolol, amlodipine, diltia-zem, isradipine, nicardipine, nifedipine, verapamil, captopril, doxazosin, prazosin, clonidine, guanfacine, methyldopa, hydralazine, minoxidil, reserpine

Common side effects:
Slowing of heart rate (bradycardia), drowsiness, dry mouth, postural hypo-tension, sexual dysfunction, dizziness, headache and *depression* are some adverse effects. *Gastrointestinal dysfunction* in the form of nausea and constipation may also be seen. Specifically, the massage therapists should remember that these clients are prone for postural hypotension and ensure that clients are well supported when they get off the massage table. Antihypertensives can cause *bronchospasm* and precipitate an *asthma* attack (This is the opposite effect of the sympathetic system that causes dilation of the bronchus). In the renal system, antihypertensives can cause *urinary retention.*

Antiinflammatories

Antiinflammatory drugs can be nonsteroidal or steroidal and the side effects vary accordingly. They are used in any condition where inflammation has to be reduced. They may be used for short or long periods according to the disease.

Nonsteroidal antiinflammatory drugs (NSAID):

examples: aspirin (acetyl salicylate), mobidin (magnesium salicylate), magan, arthropan liquid, trilisate, tylenol, dsalcid, voltaren (diclofenac sodium), dolobid (diflunisal), lodine, nalfon, ansaid, motrin, rufen (ibuprofen), indocin (indo-methacin), indocin, orudis (ketoprophen), meclomen (meclofenamate sodium), relafen, naprosyn (naproxen), anaprox, daypro (oxaprozin), butazolidin (phenyl-butazone), feldene (piroxicam), clinoril (sulindac), tolectin (tolmetin)

Common side effects:
The major side effects are related to the gastrointestinal system in the form of *nausea, indigestion* and development of *peptic ulcers.* The gastrointestinal irritation can be reduced by intake of these drugs after food or by using enteric coated drugs. All NSAIDs reduce the functioning of platelets resulting in *bleeding*

tendencies. Some people may be allergic to aspirin and the drug may produce *hypersensitivity* reactions like bronchospasm (asthma) and generalized swelling. NSAIDs can be *toxic to the kidney* and *liver* and should be used very cautiously in those with already existing renal/kidney disease.

Steroidal antiinflammatories:

These are among the most potent antiinflammatory drugs available and are used in severe inflammatory diseases like arthritis of multiple joints (eg. rheumatoid arthritis) and in those with severe, chronic symptoms (eg. SLE) or those not responding to NSAIDs. Steroids may be given orally, as injections or applied topically.

examples: glucocorticoids - hydrocortisone (cortisol), cortisone, prednisone, prednisolone, methylprednisolone, triamcinolone, paramethasone, dexamethasone, betamethasone

Common side effects:
Since the externally administered steroids are similar in structure to those secreted by the adrenal cortex, they *suppress the normal interaction between the hypothalamus, pituitary and adrenal cortex.* This adrenal suppression may present as *weight loss, lethargy, fever* and *postural hypotension* especially at the time of severe stress. In the massage clinic, postural hypotension may manifest as dizziness on getting off the table. The therapist should ensure that the client gets up slowly after a massage and is well supported while changing posture.

Steroids also suppress the immunity (*immunosuppression*) and increase the susceptibility to infection. Thus exposure to even minor local infections may manifest as a severe systemic forms. Also, infections that do not harm a normal individual may be harmful in those on steroids. The situation is made worse by the fact that steroids suppress local and systemic signs of infections such as inflammation. Infections that have been in an inactive stage - such as tuberculosis (TB) may surface as active forms when the immunity is suppressed. The massage therapist should therefore ensure that clients on steroids are not exposed to any form of disease in the clinic. Also, it should be ensured that these clients are not carriers of diseases such as TB, that may be harmful to the therapist.

Endocrine abnormalities such as *diabetes mellitus, fluid and electrolyte imbalances* characterized by edema, and hypertension are other adverse effects. The individual tends to become obese with the accumulation of fat more in the trunk (*trunkal obesity*). The face becomes rounded and fat deposition behind the neck gives the appearance of a buffalo hump.

The effect on the musculoskeletal system results in *osteoporosis.* Fractures are common in these individuals and the therapist should take care that only light pressure is used during massage. The muscles may be weak. Other adverse effects include *changes in mental status* ranging from nervousness, euphoria, insomnia to severe depression.

Antimicrobial agents

Antimicrobials are prescribed by a physician after careful consideration as they are expensive and have side effects. Also, due to the increasing incidence of resistant organisms, care is taken to prescribe an antimicrobial that has an effect on as narrow a spectrum of microorganisms as possible.

Depending on the seriousness of the infection, antimicrobials are given intravenously, intramuscularly or orally. The dosage is altered according to the condition of the person - eg. if there is associated kidney or liver disease there are chances of the drug being metabolized and excreted at a much slower rate so the dosage has to be reduced. In pregnant women, care has to be taken that the drug does not cross the placenta and affect the development of the fetus.

In general, in acute, uncomplicated infections, the duration of therapy is continued till the person has no fever for at least 72 hours. However, in complicated diseases like infections of the heart, bone and joints, treatment may have to be continued for a very long period.

Antibacterial agents:

examples: penicillins, cephalosporins, erythromycin, tetracyclines, chloramphenicol, sulphonamides, trimethoprim, metronidazole, aminoglycosides

Common side effects:
Hypersensitivity is the most common side effect of the penicillin and cephalosporin groups. If a client gives a history of hypersensitivity to penicillin it is likely that they may be allergic to other substances in addition, so special precautions should be taken while treating these clients.

The cephalosporin group may produce *inflammation of the veins* and increase the *tendency of blood to clot*. In high doses, *seizures* may occur in susceptible individuals.

Other side effects include *gastrointestinal upsets*, and with prolonged use, *candidiasis* in the oral/ vaginal mucosa. The later is due to the destruction of the microorganisms that are normally present in the body. The aminoglycosides tend to produce *toxic effects in the kidney and the inner ear* especially with prolonged use(>14 days). Hearing loss, giddiness, gait imbalance may be some of the adverse effects.

Antifungal Agents:

examples: amphotericin, flucytosine, azoles (ketoconazole, fluconazole, miconazole, itraconazole)

Common side effects:
Acute side effects include *fever, chills, headache, muscle pain, nausea* and *vomiting.* Amphoterecin which is given intravenously tends to cause *thrombophlebitis* and *renal toxicity.*

Antitubercular Agents:

Due to the higher incidence of resistance, a minimum of two drugs are given to treat tuberculosis. Also, since the bacilli takes a long time to multiply, treatment is continued over a long period (6-12 months).

examples: isoniazid (INH), rifampicin, pyrazinamide, ethambutol, streptomycin

Common side effects:
One of the adverse effects is the *hepatotoxicity* (toxicity to the liver). Hepatitis can occur especially in those who are alcoholics. *Peripheral Neuropathy* is a dose related complication of INH therapy. Care should be taken by the therapist to ensure that undue pressure is not used in these individuals as the sensations are lower in the periphery. Rarely, ethambutol can produce *inflammation of the optic nerve* leading to decreased green color perception, and diminished sight. Streptomycin can result in *inner ear problems* such as loss of hearing, gait imbalance, giddiness and ringing in the ear.

Antiviral agents:

examples: amantidine, rimantidine, acyclovir, ganciclovir, foscarnet, zidovidine

Common side effects:
In general, side effects are *uncommon.* They may be associated with *gastrointestinal complaints* such as nausea and vomiting. Some of the antifungals may cause *nephrotoxicity* (ie affect the normal functioning of the kidney).

Cancer Chemotherapy

Chemotherapy is given to treat many different types of cancer either alone or in combination with radiotherapy and/or surgery. The dosage is calculated based on the body surface area. They may be given orally, intravenously or injected directly into the affected site. They act by suppressing the rapid multiplication of cells. Since they target multiplying cells, in addition to the cancer, they tend to suppress the activity of the bone marrow, gastrointestinal tract, ovaries and testis where multiplication of normal tissue occurs.

examples: Ara-C, cytosine arabinoside, fludarabine, 5-Fluorouracil, methotrexate, busulfan, chlorambucil, cyclophosphamide, melphalan, limustine, bleomycin, dosorubicin, etoposide, vinblastine, vincristine, carboplatin, L-Asparaginase, procarbazine

Common side effects:

The most common side effects are *suppression of the bone marrow* and *toxicity to the gastrointestinal tract.* The reduction in the white blood cells make these individuals more *prone to infections.* The therapist should ensure that the clients on chemotherapy are not exposed to any form of infection in the clinic. The suppression of the platelet formation affects the clotting process, increasing the *tendency to bleed.* The therapist should therefore closely monitor the pressure used to prevent bleeding under the skin. The suppression of red blood cell formation leads to *anemia.*

The gastrointestinal effect presents as *stomatitis, diarrhea, nausea* and *vomiting.* Most of the agents produce *alopecia* (loss of hair). In general, chemotherapy agents are *toxic to almost all systems* and require careful monitoring and alteration of dosage.

In those clients where the agent is given intravenously, leak into the local tissue can produce *pain* and *redness at the injection site.* Hot /cold compresses are used to minimize the symptoms. The death of tissue at the local site may require surgery and skin grafting.

Diuretics

Diuretics are drugs that increase the excretion of water and electrolytes in the urine. They are usually given in conditions that increase the load on the heart, renal failure and edema.

examples: thiazides (chlorothiazide, benzthiazide), loop diuretics (furosemide, ethacrynic acid), spironolactone, amiloride, triamterene

Common side effects:
Diuretics can lead to *dehydration* and *electrolyte imbalances.*

Oral Contraceptives

Contraceptive pills are similar to the steroid sex hormones and are given in varying combinations and concentrations throughout the menstrual cycle. The combination and dosage of hormones are adjusted to suppress ovulation in the female while minimizing the normal cyclical secretion. The pills contain a combination of estrogen and progestogen.

examples: ortho-Novum (mestronol, norethindone combination), norinyl, ovcon, ovral, demulen, norlestrin, nordette, micronon, Nor Q.D., ovrette

Common side effects:
The incidence of *deep vein thrombosis* and *pulmonary embolism* is higher in those women using oral contraceptives. A therapist should be alert regarding symptoms

of deep vein thrombosis in these women and refer them to a physician if there is a suspicion of this. A small *increase in blood pressure* is also common. Some women may have *abnormal glucose tolerance*. Incidence of *gall stones* have been found to be higher in women on oral contraceptives. Other effects include *breast discomfort, weight gain,* development of *pigmentation of the face,* and *psychological symptoms* like depression and alteration in sexual function.

Pain killers

The best treatment for pain is to remove the cause. However, most often the cause cannot be identified easily. Therefore, analgesics (pain killers) are resorted to even before diagnosis is made.

Nonsteroidal antiinflammatory agents (NSAIDs) are most commonly used (see under antiinflammatories). These reduce pain by reducing the inflammatory reaction. Opiod analgesics are the most potent pain relievers currently available.

The opioid act on the central nervous system and activate pain-inhibitory neurons and directly inhibit neurons that transmit pain. For chronic pain as in postherpetic neuralgia, tension headache, migraine headache, chronic low back pain and cancer, antidepressant medications, anticonvulsants and antiarrythmics may be used.

examples: NSAIDs (see under antiinflammatories), opioid - codeine, oxycodone, morphine, levorphanol, methadone, meperidine, fentanyl, butorphanol; Antidepressants - doxepin, amitriptyline, imipramine, nortriptyline, dsipramine; Anticonvulsants and antiarrhythmics - phenytoin, carbamazepine, clonazepam, mexiletine

Common side effects:
For the side effects of NSAIDs see under antiinflammatories. The opiods can produce *sedation, itching, constipation* and rarely *respiratory depression*. There is a risk of *addiction* to the pain killers - especially the opioids (narcotics). Massage therapists have to obtain a detailed history of the use of pain killers as injury to the tissue may be inflicted inadvertently by excessive use of pressure in these individuals with lowered sensitivity to pain.

Radiation therapy

Radiation therapy is given to treat many types of cancer. Often it is given alone, or in combination with chemotherapy and /or surgery. Like chemotherapy, radiation suppresses rapidly multiplying cells. To reduce its effects on the bone marrow, gastrointestinal tract and the gonads (ovary and testis), radiation is targeted to local sites by shielding the normal surrounding tissue from radiation.

Common side effects:

Radiation can be *toxic to the local area*. The severity depends on the dose, location of therapy and the rate of delivery. Acute toxicity develops within the first 3 months and presents as an inflammatory reaction. This may be treated with antiinflammatories and cold compresses to the local site. The therapist should ensure that oil is not used at the radiation site as it may affect the rate of radiation delivery. By suppressing the immune cells, radiation may also make the individual more *prone to infection*. The therapist should ensure that these clients are not exposed to even mild infections in the clinic. Associated *bleeding tendencies* and anemia may also be seen. While massaging only light pressure should be used to prevent small bleeds under the skin.

Gastrointestinal toxicity can present as loss of appetite, nausea, vomiting and diarrhea. Radiation may result in subacute/chronic toxicities where fibrosis and scarring can occur at the injection site. Techniques such as transverse friction can be used to reduce adhesions.

Resources for specific disorders
(Canada & USA)

Canada

AIDS/ Sexually Transmitted Disease Information:
The AIDS Foundation of Canada
885 Dunsmuir St Suite 1000,
Vancouver BC V6C 1N5   Tel: 1 (800) 772 2437

Alcoholism:
Alcoholic Anonymous (AA)
101 128 15th Ave SW,
Calgary AB   T2R 0P5   Tel: (403) 265 8888

Allergy:
Allergy and Environmental Health Association
PO Box 40604,
Burlington ON L7P 4W1   Tel: 1 (800) 695 9271

Alzheimer's Disease:
Alzheimer Society of Canada
1320 Yonge St Suite 201,
Toronto ON M4T 1X2   Tel: (416) 925 3552 Fax: (416) 925 1649

Amyotrophic Lateral Sclerosis:
Amyotrophic Lateral Sclerosis Society of Canada
220-6 Adelaide St E,
Toronto ON M5C 1H6   Tel: (416) 362 0269 Fax: (416) 362 0414

Anemia:
Aplastic Anemia Association of Canada
22 Aikenhead Road,
Etobicoke ON M9R 2Z3   Tel: (416) 235 0468

Arthritis:
The Arthritis Society
250 Bloor St E Suite 901,
Toronto ON M4W 3P2   Tel: (416) 967 1414 Fax: (416) 967 7171

Asthma:
Asthma Society of Canada
130 Bridgeland Ave Suite 425,
Toronto ON M6A 1Z4   Tel: (416) 787 4050   Fax: (416) 787 5807

Cancer:
Cancer Information Service
755 Concession St Suite 201,
Hamilton ON L8V 1C4   Tel: (905) 387 1153 Fax: (905) 387 0376

Celiac Disease:
Canadian Celiac Association
651 9 B Mississauga Rd,
Mississauga ON L5N 1A6   Tel: (905) 567 7195 Fax: (905) 567 0710

Cerebral Palsy:
Cerebral Palsy Association of Alberta
106 5940 Macleod Tr S,
Calgary AB T2A 2G4   Tel: (403) 253 5955 Fax: (403) 258 0812

Crohn's Disease:
Crohn's and Colitis Foundation of Canada
21 St. Clair Avenue East Suite 301,
Toronto ON M4T 1L9   Tel: (416) 920 5035 or (800) 387 1479

Cystic Fibrosis:
Canadian Cystic Fibrosis Foundation
2221 Yonge St Suite 601,
Toronto ON M4S 2B4   Tel: (800) 378 2233 Fax: (416) 485 0960

Diabetes Mellitus:
Canadian Diabetes Association
15 Toronto St Suite 1101,
Toronto ON M5C 2E3   Tel: (416) 363 3373 Fax: (416) 214 1899

Epilepsy:
Epilepsy Canada
1470 Peel St Suite 745,
Montreal PQ H3A 1T1   Tel: (514) 845 7855 Fax: (514) 845 7866

Hemophilia:
Canadian Hemophilia Society
625 President Kennedy Ave Suite 1210,
Montreal PQ H3A 1K2   Tel: (514) 848 0503 Fax: (514) 848 9661

Huntington's disease:
Huntington Society of Canada
13 Water St. N Suite 3 PO Box 1269,
Cambridge ON N1R 7G6   Tel: (519) 622 1002   Fax: (519) 622 7370

Hypertension:
Canadian coalition for high blood pressure prevention and control
Stroke Research Centre U of Saskatchewan,
Saskatoon S7N 0W0   Tel: (306) 966 7695 Fax: (306) 966 7685

Infectious Diseases:
Canadian Infectious Disease Society
c/o Hospital Saint - Luc 1058 rue Saint Denis St.,
Montreal ON H2X 3J4   Tel: (514) 281 2100 Fax: (514) 281 2443

Lupus Erythematosus:
Lupus Canada
Box 64034 5512   4th Street NW,
Calgary AB T2K 6J1
          Tel: (403) 274 5599 or (800) 661 1468 Fax: (403) 274 5599

Multiple Sclerosis:
Multiple Sclerosis Society of Canada
250 Bloor St E Suite 1000,
Toronto ON M4W 3P9   Tel: (416) 922 6065 Fax: (416) 922 7538

Muscular Dystrophy:
Muscular Dystrophy Association of Canada
2345 Yonge St Suite 900,
Toronto ON M4P 2E5
          Tel: (416) 488 0030 or (800) 567 2873 Fax: (416) 488 7523

Myasthenia Gravis:
Myasthenia Gravis Association
2805 Kingsway,
Vancouver BC V5R 5H9   Tel: (604) 451 5511 Fax: (604) 451 5651

Neurofibromatosis:
Neurofibromatosis Society of Ontario
923 Annes St,
Whitby ON L1N 5K7   Tel: (905) 430 6141 Fax: (905) 430 6141

Parkinsons's disease:
Parkinson's Society of Southern Alberta.
480D 36th Avenue SE
Calgary Alberta T2G 1W4   Tel: (403) 243 9901 Fax: (403) 243 8283

Psoriasis:
Canadian Psoriasis Foundation
1306 Wellington Street Suite 500 A,
Ottawa ON K1Y 3B2
                    Tel: (613) 728 4000 or (800) 265 0926 Fax: (613) 728 8913

Spina Bifida:
Spina Bifida Association of Canada
388 Donald St Suite 220,
Winnipeg MB R3B 2J4
                    Tel: (204) 957 1784 or (800) 565 9488 Fax: (204) 957 1794

Ulcerative Colitis:
Crohn's and Colitis Foundation of Canada,
21 St Clair Avenue East Suite 301,
Toronto Ontario M4T 1L9   Tel: 1(416) 920 5035 or 1(800) 387 1479

Miscellaneous:
The Health Connection, Calgary   Tel: (403) 571 8070

Alberta Massage Therapy Association
PO Box 24031,
Red Deer AB T4N 6X6   Tel: (403) 340 1913 Fax: (403) 346 2269

USA

AIDS/ Sexually Transmitted Disease Information:
Body Positive
19 Fulton St Ste 308B,
New York NY 10038

Tel: (212) 566 7333 Fax: (212) 566 4539

Alcoholism:
Alcoholics Anonymous(AA) World Services
PO Box 459 Grand Central Station,
NewYork NY 10163   Tel: (212) 870 3400

Allergy:
American Allergy Association
PO Box 7273 Menlo Park,
CA 94026   Tel: (415) 855 8036

Alzheimer's Disease:
Alzheimer's Association
919 N Michigan Ave Ste 1000,
Chicago IL 60611   Tel: (312) 335 8700 or (800) 272 3900 Fax: (312) 335 1110

Amyotrophic Lateral Sclerosis:
Amyotrophic Lateral Sclerosis Association
21021 Ventura Bld Ste 321,
Woodland Hills CA 91364   Tel: (818) 340 7500 or (800) 782 4747

Anorexia Nervosa:
Anorexia Nervosa and Related Eating Disorders
PO Box 5102,
Eugene OR 97405   Tel: (541) 344 1144

Arthritis:
Arthritis Foundation
1314 Spring St NW,
Atlanta GA 30329   Tel: (800) 283 7800

Asthma:
Asthma and Allergy Foundation of America
1125 15th St NW Ste 502,
Washington DC 20005
Tel: (202) 466 7643 or (800) 7 ASTHMA Fax: (202) 466 8940

Cancer:
American Association for Cancer Education
MD Anderson Cancer Centre
Department of Epidemiology 1515 Holocombe Blvd,
Houston TX 77030   Tel: (713) 792 3020 Fax: (713) 792 0807

Cancer Information Service
Office of Cancer Communication
NCI/NIH Bldg 31 10A07 31 Center Dr MSC 2580,
Bethesda MD 20892-2580   Tel: (800) 4 CANCER Fax: (301) 402 0555

National Alliance of Breast Cancer Organisations
9E 37th St 10th Floor,
NewYork NY 10016
              Tel: (212) 719 0154 or (800) 719 9154 Fax: (212) 689 1213

Celiac Disease:
Celiac disease Foundation
13251 Ventura Blvd Ste 3,
Studio City CA 91604 1838   Tel: (818) 990 2354 Fax: (818) 990 2379

Cerebral Palsy:
United Cerebral Palsy Association
1660 L St NW Suite 700
Washington DC 20036   Tel: (202) 842 1266 Fax: (202) 776 0414

Chronic Fatigue Syndrome:
CFIDS
PO Box 220398,
Charlotte NC 28222 0398   Tel: (800) 442 3437 or (704) 365 9755

Crohn's Disease:
Crohn's and Colitis Foundation of America
386 Park Ave S,
New York NY 10016 8804
              Tel: (212) 685 3440 or (800) 932 2423 Fax: (212) 779 4098

Cystic Fibrosis:
Cystic Fibrosis Foundation
6931 Arlington Rd Suite 200,
Bethesda MD 20814   Tel: (800) 344 4823

Diabetes Mellitus:
American Association of Diabetes Educators
444 N Michigan Ave Ste 1240,
Chicago IL 60611 3901
                    Tel: (312) 644 2233 or (800) 338 DMED Fax: (312) 644 4411

American Diabetes Association
1660 Duke St,
Alexandria VA 22314   Tel: (800) 232 3472

Juvenile Diabetes Foundation International
120 Wall St. 19th Floor
New York NY 10005   Tel: 1 (800) 223 1138

Eczema:
Eczema Association for Science and Education
1221 SW Yamhill No 303,
Portland OR 97205   Tel: (503) 228 4430 Fax: (503) 273 8778

Fibromyalgia:
National Chronic Fatigue Syndrome and Fibromyalgia Association
3521 Broadway Ste 222,
Kansas City MO 64111   Tel: (816) 931 4777 Fax: (816) 524 6782

Guillain-Barre Syndrome:
Guillain-Barre Syndrome Foundation International
PO Box 262,
Wynnewood PA 19096   Tel: (610) 667 0131 Fax: (610) 667 7036

Headache:
National Headache Foundation
5252 N Western Ave,
Chicago IL 60625   Tel: (312) 388 6399 or (800) 843 2256 Fax: (312) 907 6278

Hemophilia:
National Hemophilia Foundation
110 GreeneSt Ste 303,
New York NY 10012   Tel: (212) 219 8180 Fax: (212) 431 0906

Huntington's Disease:
Huntington's Disease Society of America
140 W 22nd St 6th Floor,
NewYork NY 10011   Tel: (800) 345 4372

Hypertension:
American Society of Hypertension
515 Madison Ave Ste 1212,
New York NY 10022   Tel: (212) 644 0650 Fax: (212) 644 0658

Infectious Disease:
Centers for Infectious Disease Control
1600 Clifton Rd NE,
Atlanta GA 30333   Tel: (404) 639 3534 or (404) 639 3535

National Vaccine Information Center
512 Maple Ave W Ste 206,
Vienna VA 22180
              Tel: (703) 938 DPT3 or (800) 909 SHOT Fax: (703) 938 5768

Leukemia:
Leukemia Society of America
600 3rd Ave,
New York NY 10016
              Tel: (212) 573 8484 or (800) 955 4LSA Fax: (212) 856 9686

Lupus Erythematosis:
Lupus Foundation of America
1300 Piccard Dr. Suite 200
Rockville MD 20850 3226
              Tel: (301) 670 9292 or (800) 558 0121 Fax: (301) 670 9486

Multiple Sclerosis:
National Multiple Sclerosis Society
733 Third Ave 6th Floor,
New York NY 10017   Tel: (800)344 4867

Muscular Dystrophy:
Muscular Dystrophy Association
3300E Sunrise Dr,
Tuscon AZ 85718   Tel: (602) 529 2000 Fax: (520) 529 5300

Myasthenia Gravis:
Myasthenia Gravis Association
222 S Riverside Plaza Suite 1540,
Chicago IL 60606   Tel: (800) 541 5454 Fax (312) 258 0461

Myeloma:
International Myeloma Foundation
2120 Stanley Hills Dr
Los Angeles CA 90046   Tel: (800) 452 CURE   Fax: (213) 656 1182

Neuralgia:
Trigeminal Neuralgia Association
PO Box 785, Barnegat Light
NJ 08006   Tel: (609) 361 1014   Fax: (609) 361 0982

Neurofibromatosis:
Neurofibromatosis Inc.
8855 Annapolis Rd Ste 110,
Lahnam MD 20706 2924
           Tel: (301) 577 8984 or (800) 942 6825 Fax: (301) 577 0016

Paralysis/ Stroke:
American Paralysis Association
500 Morris Ave,
Springfield NJ 07081
           Tel: (201) 379 2690 or (800) 225 0292 Fax: (201) 914 9433
Stroke Clubs International
805 12 St,
Galveston TX 77550   Tel: (409) 762 1022

Parkinson's Disease:
American Parkinson's Disease Association
1250 Hylan Blvd Ste B4,
Staten Island NY 10305
           Tel: (718) 981 8001 or (800) 223 2132 Fax: (718) 981 4399

National Parkinson's Foundation
1501 NW 9th Ave,
Miami FL 33136   Tel: (305) 547 6666 Fax: (305) 243 4403

Poliomyelitis:
International Polio Network
4207 Lindell Blvd No.110,
St Louis MO 63108   Tel: (314) 534 0475 Fax: (314) 534 5070

Psoriasis:
National Psoriasis Foundation
6600 SW 92nd Ave Suite 300
Portland OR 97223 7195
           Tel: (503) 244 7404 or (800) 723 9166 Fax: (503) 245 0626

Scleroderma:
Scleroderma Federation
Peabody Office Bldg 1 Newbury St,
Peabody MA 01960
                    Tel: (508) 535 6600 or (800) 422 1113 Fax: (508) 535 6696

Scoliosis:
National Scoliosis Foundation
72 Mt Auburn St,
Waterton MA 02172   Tel: (617) 341 6333 Fax: (617) 341 8333

Spina Bifida:
Spina Bifida Association of America
5 Cabot Place,
Stoughton, Masachusets 02072   Tel: (800) 621 3141

Miscellaneous:
American Massage Therpay Association
820 Danns St Ste 100,
Evanston IL 60201 4444   Tel: (847) 864 0123 Fax: (847) 864 1178

Committee for Freedom of Choice in Medicine
1180 Walnut Ave,
Chula Vista CA 91911
                    Tel: (619) 429 8200 or (800) 227 4473 Fax: (619) 429 8004

Alliance for Alternatives in Health Care
PO Box 6279, Thousand Oaks,
CA 91359 6279   Tel: (805) 494 7818 Fax: (805) 494 8528

National Association for Holistic Aromatherapy
PO Box 17622,
Boulder CO 80308 7622
                    Tel: (415) 564 6785 or (800) 566 6735 Fax: (415) 564 6799

Rieki Alliance
PO Box 41,
Calaldo ID 83810   Tel: (208) 682 3535 Fax: (208) 682 4848

Touch for Health Association
6955 Fernhill Dr Ste 5A
Malibu CA 90 265 4238
                    Tel: (310) 574 7833 or (800) 466 TFHA Fax: (310) 457 9267

Key references

Beck WJ, Davies JE: Medical Parasitology. 3rd ed. London, Mosby Company, 1981.

Bluefarb SM: Dermatology. Michigan, UpJohn Company, 1978.

Ewald GA, McKenzie CR: Manual of Medical Therapeutics. 28th ed. London, Little, Brown & Company, 1995.

Farrar WE, Wood MJ, Innes JA, Tubbs H: Infectious diseases text and color atlas. 2nd ed. London, Gower Medical Publishing, 1992.

Hay RJ: Common Bacterial Infections of the Skin. Distributed by Leo Laboratories Canada Ltd.

Hertling D, Kessler RM: Manual of common musculoskeletal disorders - physical therapy principals and methods. 3rd ed. Philadelphia, Lippincott company, 1996.

Isselbacher KJ, Braunwald E, Wilson JD, Martin JB, Fauci AS, Kasper DL: Harrison's principles of internal medicine. 13th ed. London, McGraw-Hill Inc., 1994.

Joan J: The healing art of sports massage. Pennsylvania, Rodale Press Inc., 1995.

Lawrence RM, Rosenberg S: Pain Relief with Osteomassage. California, Woodbridge Press, 1982.

Massage Magazine: various volumes.

Melzack R, Wall P: The challenge of pain. New York, Penguin Books, 1988.

Mosby's Medical, Nursing & Allied Health Dictionary. 4th ed. St Louis, Missouri, Mosby Year Book Inc., 1994.

Newton D: Pathology for Massage therapists. 2nd ed. Oregon, Simran publications, 1995.

Professional guide to diseases. 5th ed. Pennsylvania, Springhouse corporation, 1995.

Porth CM: Pathophysiology concepts of altered health states. 4th ed. Philadelphia, Lippincott company, 1994.

Rattray FS: Massage Therapy - An approach to treatments. 1st ed. Toronto,

Massage Therapy Texts and MAVerick Consultants, 1994.

Schaffer SD, Garzon LS, Heroux DL, Korniewicz DM: Infection Prevention and Safe Practice. London, Mosby Year Book Inc, 1996.

Sexually Transmitted Diseases. Alberta Health, 1995.

Shulman ST, Phair JP, Sommers HM: The biologic & clinical basis of Infectious Diseases. 4th ed. Philadelphia, WB Saunders Company, 1992.

Sparatto GR, Woods AL: Nurse's Drug Reference. New York, Delmar Publishers, 1995.

Stein AM, Jacobson NH: NCLEX-RN Review. New York, Delmar Publishers, 1992.

Van De Graaff KM, Fox SI: Concepts of Human Anatomy and Physiology. 4th ed. London, Wm C Brown Publishers, 1995.

Wale JO: Tidy's massage and remedial exercises. 11th ed. Bristol, John Wright & Sons Ltd, 1968.

Martini FH: Fundamentals of Anatomy and Physiology. 3rd ed. New Jersey, Prentice Hall, 1995.

Glossary

A

abduction to move a body part away from the midline of the body; to move digits away from the axis of limb

abscess a cavity containing pus, surrounded by inflamed tissue

adduction to move a body part towards the midline of the body; to move digits towards the axis of the limb

acute disease disease beginning suddenly/abruptly, and subsiding after a short period

agonist a muscle that produces the same movement as another muscle

allergy a state of hypersensitivity caused by exposure to an antigen. It causes histamine and other molecules to be liberated in the site by the action of the immune system

alveoli grapelike, thin sacs in the lungs, which are surrounded by blood vessels, where exchange of oxygen and carbon-di-oxide takes place

antagonist a muscle that opposes the movement of another muscle

antibodies proteins secreted by B lymphocytes that target specific antigens

antigen a molecule - usually a protein, that triggers the production of antibodies

arteriosclerosis any one of a group of diseases that cause the wall of arteries to thicken and harden

artery a blood vessel that carries blood *away* from the heart

articulation a joint

atrium the right/left chamber of the heart that *receives* blood from the veins

atrophy a decrease in the size of a cell/tissue/organ

autoimmune immunity acting against self

autonomic nervous system the part of the nervous system that controls the internal organs and skin; consists of the sympathetic and parasympathetic systems

B

baroreceptor nerve receptors that monitor the pressure in the blood vessels

basal ganglia a collection of gray mater located near the center of the brain; responsible for stability and coordinated movement

benign not malignant; used in reference to tumors that increase very slowly in size and do not spread

bile secretion from the liver that is stored in the gall bladder and released into the gut through the common bile duct

bilirubin a pigment that is a breakdown product of hemoglobin

B lymphocytes a type of white blood cells that produce antibodies

brain stem part of the central nervous system that lies between the spinal cord and the brain; includes the medulla oblongata, pons and midbrain

bronchus a branch of the trachea that conducts air into the lungs

bullae a large fluid-filled lesion

bursa a synovial fluid-filled sac which serves to reduce friction between muscle and joints/ muscle and muscle/ skin and muscle/ bone and muscle

C

calcitonin a hormone secreted by certain cells in the thyroid gland; it helps to *reduce* calcium levels in the blood

cancer a tumor characterized by abnormal and rapidly multiplying cells; usually refers to malignant tumors

capillary the smallest blood vessel that allows exchange of substances; it connects an arteriole with a venule

cartilage a type of connective tissue that has more elastic matrix and less calcium than bone

cecum a pouchlike area that lies at the junction of the small intestine and ascending colon

cell the smallest structure of the body that is capable of performing all the functions necessary for life

central nervous system part of the nervous system which includes the brain and the spinal cord

cerebellum part of the brain involved with the coordination of the skeletal muscles

cerebrospinal fluid circulating fluid that fills the ventricles of the brain, surrounds and bathes the brain and spinal cord

cervix the narrow necklike portion of an organ; in the uterus it is the part that projects into the vagina

chromosomes structures in the nucleus of a cell that contain the genes

chronic disease developing slowly and lasting for a long time

cilia thin thread-like projections that are present in certain epithelial cells

coagulation clotting of blood

concussion a violent jarring of the brain caused by a sudden change in momentum.

congenital present at the time of birth

congestion abnormal accumulation of fluid in an area

consolidation a process of becoming solid

connective tissue binding and supportive tissue

contagious a disease that is communicable - spread from one person to another

contracture an abnormal permanent contraction of a muscle which can occur in paralyzed muscle

coronary circulation the arterial and venous circulation that supply the walls of the heart

cyanosis blue discoloration of the mucous membranes due to excess of deoxygenated hemoglobin

D

deep towards the core of the body

degeneration the slow death/deterioration of cells

dementia a chronic mental disease

dendrite a process of the neuron that conducts impulses towards the cell body of the neuron

dermis the inner layer of the skin where the glands, nerve endings and blood vessels are located

diastole the period of the cardiac cycle when the chambers are relaxed

distal away from the trunk

diuretic an agent that promotes excretion of urine

dorsal refers to the posterior portion of a body part

dorsiflexion movement of the ankle where the dorsum is elevated

dyspnea *subjective* difficulty in breathing

E

effleurage a massage technique where broad, light or firm strokes are used

electrolytes ions and molecules that can carry positive or negative electric charges

endemic refers to the presence of a disease in the local population or geographical area

endocrine gland a gland without ducts that secretes hormones directly into the blood

epidemic refers to the spread of disease rapidly through a population affecting a large number of people at the same time

epidermis the superficial layer of the skin

epithelium type of tissue that lines or covers body surfaces

estrogens any of the many hormones secreted by the follicles of the ovary

eversion a movement of the foot where the sole of the foot faces outwards

exacerbation an increase in the severity of the disease

extension a movement that results in an increase in the angle between the parts of a joint

external located on or towards the body surface

extravasation escape of fluid (usually blood) into the tissues

F

fascia a tough sheet of fibrous connective tissue that surrounds/ supports muscles or binds skin to underlying muscle

fetus a prenatal human after 8 weeks of pregnancy

flexion a movement that decreases the angle between the parts of a joint

G

gall bladder a sac lying beneath the liver that stores bile

ganglion a collection of the cell bodies of nerve cells outside the central nervous system

glans penis the enlarged distal, sensitive portion of the penis

glomerulus a tuft of capillaries that are surrounded by a cup-shaped capsule that filters urine from the blood, in the kidney

H

hemoglobin the (iron containing protein) pigment in the red blood cell responsible for carrying oxygen and carbon dioxide

hormone a chemical secreted by an endocrine gland into the blood; it causes an effect in a specified organ *away* from the site of origin of the hormone

hyperplasia an increase in the size of the organ due to an increase in the *number* of cells

hypertrophy increase in the size of organ due to increase in *size* of individual cells

hypoxia a low concentration of oxygen in the blood

I

ileum   the last portion of the small intestine that connects the jejunum with the cecum

immunization   the process of increasing the resistance of the body to pathogens

incidence   the number of new cases that appear in a particular period of time

incontinence   inability to control urination or defecation

incubation period   the period between the exposure to the disease and the onset of disease

inflammation   a local reaction of the body to cell injury characterized by redness, swelling, pain, increase in temperature and loss of function

inoculation   to introduce a substance into the body through the skin

insertion   the place where the muscle is attached; indicates the part that is most mobile (opposite of origin)

interstitial compartment   the fluid space between the cells but outside the blood and lymph vessels

intervertebral disc   the cartilage that lies between two vertebrae

inversion   a movement where the sole of the foot is turned inwards

ischemia   an inadequate supply of oxygen to the tissue

isometric   muscle contraction in which there is no lengthening of muscle fibres but an increase in tension occurs

isotonic   muscle contraction in which there is lengthening of muscle fibres and the same amount of tension is maintained

J

jejunum   part of the small intestine that lies between the duodenum and ileum

L

labia   a part of the external genitalia of the female consisting of two longitudinal folds that extend inferiorly and posteriorly; two pairs labia majora and labia minora are present

large intestine   part of the gastrointestinal tract that includes the cecum, colon, rectum and anal canal

latent   a period when the infection is lying dormant

lateral   towards the side of the body

lesion   a wounded or damaged area

leukocyte   white blood cell; includes eosinophils, basophils, neutrophils, lymphocytes and monocytes

ligament a tough cord or band that binds bone to bone

lumen the space within a tubular structure through which substances pass

lymph the fluid that flows through the lymph vessels

lymph node an oval mass with a collection of lymphocytes through which the lymph pass

lymphocyte a type of white blood cell involved in immunity; constitutes 20-25% of all white blood cells

M

macrophage a large white blood cell capable of phagocytosis

macule an irregular lesion not raised on the surface of the skin

malignant virulent; refers to a tumor that grows and spreads at a rapid rate

mast cell a cell found in the connective tissue that secretes histamine and participates in local inflammation

medial closer or towards the midline of the body

meninges the fibrous membrane that covers the brain; consists of three membranes - the dura, arachnoid and pia mater

meniscus wedge-shaped cartilage that is found in certain types of synovial joints eg. knee

menopause the period when a female ceases to have menstrual cycle

menstruation the discharge of blood and tissue from the uterus in the first few days of the menstrual cycle; the first day of bleeding is considered day 1

metabolism the chemical changes that occur in a cell

metastasis spread from one organ or body part to another; usually refers to a malignant tumor

monocyte a white blood cell that is capable of phagocytosis; forms 3-8% of all white cells

mucosa mucous membrane that lines cavities and tubes that are exposed to the external environment

myelin a lipoprotein substance that covers nerve fibres

myocardium the muscle layer of the heart

myoneural junction the contact area between the motor nerve and the muscle

N

necrosis cell or tissue death

neoplasm a new abnormal growth

neurotransmitters a chemical stored in nerve endings that is released in the synapses; it enables communication across neurons

neutrophil a type of white blood cell that is capable of phagocytosis; it constitutes about 60-70% of all white blood cells.

O

oncotic pressure the osmotic pressure produced by proteins; in the plasma it helps counteract the tendency of the capillary hydrostatic pressure to push fluids into the interstitial space

origin the place where the muscle is attached; indicates the part that is stationary (opposite of insertion)

ossification the development of bone

ovarian follicle the developing ovum along with the surrounding epithelial cells in the ovary

P

palmar relates to the palm of the hand

pancreas a gland that secretes enzymes into the intestines; it also has an endocrine component that secretes insulin and glucagon into the blood

paranasal sinus a chamber filled with air and lined with mucous membrane that communicates with the nasal cavity

parasympathetic part of the autonomic nervous system that opposes the effect of the sympathetic system in general

paralysis loss of muscle function and/or sensation

parathyroids endocrine glands located posterior to the thyroid glands that secrete parathormone; regulates calcium metabolism

pericardium a membrane that surrounds the heart

peritoneum the membrane that lines the abdominal cavity and covers the abdominal organs

petrissage a massage stroke where the skin is lifted and squeezed as in kneading

pH a measure of the acidity/alkalinity of a solution; ranges from 0-14, with 7 denoting neutral and 7+ to 14 denoting the alkalinity

phagocytosis the ability of certain white blood cells to engulf and digest large particles

placenta the organ that helps transport nutrients/ oxygen from mother to fetus

plantar sole of foot

plasma the fluid in the blood which remains after the removal of cells

platelets small fragments of certain cells in the bone marrow which primarily take part in the clotting of blood

pleural cavity   a potential cavity found between the two layers of the pleura of the lungs

polydipsia excessive thirst

polyuria passage of excessive urine

polyphagia excessive hunger

popliteal the region behind the knee

posterior towards the back

prognosis prediction of the probable outcome of the disease

prolapse an abnormal protrusion of an organ

pronation the movement that turns the palm of the hand towards the back

prostate a gland located below the urinary bladder, surrounding the male urethra

proximal closer to the core of the body

pruritus itching

psychosis a major mental disorder

R

rectum   the part of the gastrointestinal tract that lies between the colon and the anus

remission a decrease in the seriousness of the illness

rotated to move around an axis

S

sebaceous gland   a gland located near a hair follicle that secretes sebum (responsible for the oil on the skin)

serum plasma of the blood without the substances that cause clotting

sign an objective finding made by the examiner

spastic uncontrolled contraction of a muscle

spleen large blood filled organ located in the upper left quadrant of the abdomen

sputum   secretion from the lungs

stasis stagnation of fluid movement

subluxation a partial separation of the articulating surface of one bone of a joint from the other

superficial near the surface

superior above; towards the upper part

supination the movement that turns the palm upward/ anterior

sympathetic part of the autonomic system that is responsible for the 'fight or flight' reaction

symptom a subjective perception of a disease by the person with the disease

synovial cavity space between the bones of a synovial joint; filled with synovial fluid

synovial joint a freely movable joint that is lined by synovial membrane, having a synovial cavity

systole the period of the cardiac cycle when the chamber of the heart contracts

systolic pressure the blood pressure that is recorded inside an artery when the ventricle contracts

T

T cell type of lymphocyte that is responsible for the type of immunity mediated by cells

tender points painful spots usually located in the muscle

tendon tough cord-like connective tissue that connects muscle to bone

thalamus an oval grey area in the brain that serves as the sensory relay station

thrombus a blood clot formed inside a blood vessel

thymus an organ located posterior to the sternum which is part of the lymphatic system

trigger points points on the surface of the body that is very sensitive to touch

trunk the thorax and abdomen together

topical to apply on the surface of the skin

U

umbilicus the site where the umbilical cord was attached in the fetus (navel)

ureter the tube connecting the kidney to the urinary bladder

urethra the tube that transports the urine to the exterior from the bladder

V

vasoconstriction narrowing of the lumen of a blood vessel by contraction of the smooth muscles

vasodilation widening of the lumen of a blood vessel by relaxation of the smooth muscles

vasomotor center a collection of cell bodies in the brain stem responsible for regulating blood pressure

vesicle a fluid filled lesion

vein a blood vessel that carries blood *to* the heart

ventral towards the front; anterior

viscera organs inside the abdominal/thoracic cavity

vulva refers to the external genitalia of the female

Index (disease-wise)

Arthropathy, 25
Arthrosis temporomandibularis - *see* Temporomandibular joint dysfunction
    syndrome, 258
Aspergillosis - *see* Fungal infections, 111
Asthma - bronchial, 25
Atelectasis, 27
Atherosclerosis, 28

B

Basedow's disease - *see* Hyperthyroidism, 148
Becker's Dystrophy - *see* Muscular Dystrophy, 180
Bed sores - *see* Decubitus Ulcers, 80
Bell's palsy, 29
Beryllium disease - *see* Pneumoconiosis - Berylliosis, 212
Beryllium poisoning - *see* Pneumoconiosis - Berylliosis, 212
Blacklung disease - *see* Pneumoconiosis - Coal Worker's, 213
Boil - *see* Furunculitis, 112
Brittle bones - *see* Osteogenesis Imperfecta, 193
Bronchiectasis, 30
Bronchitis, 32
Bronchogenic Carcinoma, 47
Burger's disease, 33
Burns, 35
Bursitis, 36
Bursitis - iliopectineal, 37
Bursitis - prepatellar, 38
Bursitis - subdeltoid, 38
Bursitis - trochanteric, 39

C

Calcific tendinitis - rotator cuff - see Adhesive Capsulitis, 6
Cancer - bladder, 40
Cancer - breast, 41
Cancer - cervix, 43
Cancer - colon, 44
Cancer - gallbladder, 45
Cancer - kidney, 44
Cancer - liver, 46
Cancer - lung, 47
Cancer - oral, 48
Cancer - ovary, 49
Cancer - pancreas, 50
Cancer - prostate, 51
Cancer - skin, 52

D

E

F

G

H

I

N

O

P

R

S

T

U

V

W

Warts, 290
Whiplash, 291
Wry neck - *see* Torticollis, 275

Y

Yuppie flu - *see* Chronic Fatigue syndrome, 64

Word Index

Allergy *see* Hay fever, Asthma, Contact Dermatitis
Amebic dysentery *see* Dysentery
aplastic anemia *see* Anemia
Appalacian Mountain disease *see* Fungal infections
ascites *see* Cancer - liver, Esophageal varices, Portal Hypertension, Cirrhosis
Athlete's foot *see* Ringworm
Atrial Septal Defect *see* Congential heart disease

Bacillary dysentery *see* Dysentery
Basal cell Epithelioma *see* Cancer - skin
Blastomycosis *see* Fungal infections
body lice *see* Pediculosis
Brudzinski's sign *see* Meningitis

Celiac Disease *see* Malabsorption syndrome
Celiac sprue *see* Malabsorption syndrome
Central Mississippi Valley disease *see* Fungal infections
cervical rib *see* Thoracic outlet syndrome
Chlamydia *see* Pelvic Inflammatory Disease, Salpingitis
Chronic Obstructive Pulmonary Disease *see* Asthma, Bronchitis, Emphysema
Chylothorax *see* Pleural Effusion
Coarctation of Aorta *see* Congential heart disease
complete abortion *see* abortion
congenital adrenal hyperplasia *see* Adrenogenital syndrome
COPD *see* Asthma, Bronchitis, Emphysema
Costoclavicular syndrome *see* Thoracic outlet syndrome
Crabs *see* Pediculosis
Cryptococcosis *see* Fungal infections

Darling's disease *see* Fungal infections
deep vein thrombosis *see* Venous Thrombosis
disc prolapse *see* Sciatic nerve lesions

dissecting aneurysm *see* Aneurysm

Eczema *see* Contact Dermatitis
ELISA *see* Acquired Immunodeficiency Syndrome
Empyema *see* Pleural Effusion
European Blastomycosis *see* Fungal infections
exophthalmus *see* Hyperthyroidism

folic acid deficiency *see* Anemia
foot drop *see* Sciatic nerve lesions

Gilchrist's disease *see* Fungal infections
habitual abortion *see* abortion
Hamburger disease see Diarrhea
head lice *see* Pediculosis
hematemisis *see* Esophageal Varices, Portal Hypertension
hematuria *see* Renal stones
hemiplegia *see* Stroke
Hemothorax *see* Pleural Effusion
herniated disc *see* Sciatic nerve lesions
Histoplasmosis *see* Fungal infections
HIV *see* Acquired Immunodeficiency Syndrome
Hofman's sign *see* Venous Thrombosis
Hypernephroma *see* Cancer - kidney

incomplete abortion *see* abortion
inevitable abortion *see* abortion
insomnia *see* Sleep apnea
Intussusception *see* Intestinal Obstruction
iron deficiency anemia *see* Anemia

jock itch *see* Ringworm
Juvenile onset diabetes *see* Diabetes

Kernig's sign *see* Meningitis

lactose intolerance *see* Carbohydrate intolerance
lumbar sympathectomy *see* Burger's Disease

Malignant melanoma *see* Cancer - skin
Mantoux test *see* Tuberculosis
Maturity onset diabetes *see* Diabetes
melena *see* Peptic Ulcer
metastatic carcinoma *see* Cancer - liver
missed abortion *see* abortion

Nephroblastoma *see* Cancer - kidney
Nerve entrapment *see* Thoracic outlet syndrome, carpal tunnel syndrome
North American Blastomycosis *see* Fungal infections

Ohio Valley disease *see* Fungal infections
Orthostatic Hypotension *see* Hypotension
otitis media *see* Common cold

Pap smear *see* Cancer - cervix
Para coccidioidomycosis *see* Fungal infections
Paralytic ileus *see* Intestinal Obstruction
paraplegia *see* Spinal cord injury
Patent ductus arteriosus *see* Congential heart disease
Pectoralis syndrome *see* Thoracic outlet syndrome
pernicious anemia *see* Anemia
Phalen test *see* Carpal tunnel syndrome
phantom limb pain *see* Amputation
Cardiovascular system
piriformis spasm *see* Sciatic nerve lesions
polycythemia *see* Pulmonary embolism
Postural Hypotension *see* Hypotension
Pulmonary stenosis *see* Congenital heart disease
pyloric stenosis *see* Peptic Ulcer

quadriplegia *see* Spinal cord injury

Renal cell carcinoma *see* Cancer - kidney

San Joaquin Valley fever *see* Fungal infections
Scalene anterior syndrome *see* Thoracic outlet syndrome
sclerodactylia *see* Scleroderma
septic abortion *see* abortion
Sexually Transmitted Disease *see* Gonorrhea, Syphilis, AIDS, Herpes simplex,
    Warts, Scabies, Hepatitis, Pelvic inflammatory disease, Pediculosis
STD *see* Gonorrhea, Syphilis, AIDS, Herpes simplex, Warts, Scabies, Hepatitis,
Pelvic inflammatory disease, Pediculosis
sickle cell anemia *see* Anemia
slipped disc *see* Sciatic nerve lesions
spasticity *see* Spinal cord injury
spinal shock *see* Spinal cord injury
Squamous cell carcinoma *see* Cancer - skin

Tetrology of Fallot *see* Congenital heart disease
threatened abortion *see* abortion
thrombophlebitis *see* Varicos Veins
thrombus *see* Venous Thrombosis

tinea corporis *see* Ringworm
tinea cruris *see* Ringworm
tinea manus *see* Ringworm
tinea pedis *see* Ringworm
tinea unguium *see* Ringworm
Tinel's sign *see* Carpal tunnel syndrome
Torulosis *see* Fungal infections
Tubal pregnancy *see* Ectopic pregnancy
Tuberculin skin test *see* Tuberculosis

Valley fever *see* Fungal infections
VD *see* Gonorrhea, Syphilis, AIDS, Herpes simplex, Warts, Scabies, Hepatitis, Pelvic inflammatory disease, Pediculosis
Ventricular Septal Defect *see* Congenital heart disease
Venereal diseases *see* Gonorrhea, Syphilis, AIDS, Herpes simplex, Warts, Scabies, Hepatitis, Pelvic inflammatory disease, Pediculosis
Viral Hepatitis *see* Hepatitis
vitamin B12 deficiency *see* Anemia
Volvulus *see* Intestinal Obstruction

Wilm's tumor *see* Cancer - kidney

Index (system-wise)

Cardiovascular system

Endocrine system

Gastrointestinal system

Integumentary system

Tinea - see Ringworm, 231
Tinea Versicolor, 273
Varicella - see Chicken pox, 62
Veruca vulgaris - see Warts, 290
Vitiligo, 288
Von Recklinghausen's disease - see Neurofibromatosis, 183
Warts, 290

Lymphatic system

Acquired Immuno Deficiency Syndrome, 4
AIDS - see Acquired Immuno Deficiency Syndrome, 4
Edema, 90
Elephantiasis - see Filariasis, 107
Filariasis, 107
Hodgekin's Disease, 141
Human Immunodeficiency Virus Infection
        - see Acquired Immunodeficiency Syndrome, 4
Lyme arthritis - see Lyme disease, 170
Lymphangitis, 171
Lymphoma - Hodgekin's - see Hodgekin's disease, 141
Lymphosarcoma - see Malignant Lymphomas, 173
Malignant Lymphoma, 173
Non-Hodgekin's Lymphoma, 173
Oedema - see Edema, 90
Phthisis - see Tuberculosis, 280

Musculoskeletal system

Acceleration deceleration injury - see Whiplash, 291
Acromioclavicular arthritis - see Adhesive Capsulitis, 6
Adhesive Capsulitis, 6
Amputation, 11
Ankylopoietica - see Ankylosing spondylitis, 17
Ankylosing Spondylitis, 17
Anterior compartment syndrome, 18
Anterior talofibular or Calcaneocuboid ligament injury, 247
Arthritis - gouty, 20
Arthritis - infective, 21
Arthritis - osteoarthritis, 22
Arthritis - rheumatoid, 23
Arthropathy, 25
Arthrosis temporomandibularis - see Temporomandibular joint dysfunction
        syndrome, 258
Becker's Dystrophy - see Muscular Dystrophy, 180

Nervous system

Renal system

Neurofibromata - see Neurofibromatosis, 183
Neurofibromatosis, 183
Neuromatosis - see Neurofibromatosis, 183
NF - see Neurofibromatosis, 183
Oedema - see Edema, 90
Phthisis - see Tuberculosis, 280
Renal calculi - see Renal stones, 228
Pneumoconiosis - Berylliosis, 212
Renal failure, 227
Renal stones, 228
SLE - see Systemic Lupus Erythematosus, 257
Systemic Lupus Erythematosus, 257
TB - see Tuberculosis, 280
Tuberculosis, 280
Urinary tract infection, 283
Von Recklinghausen's disease - see Neurofibromatosis, 183

Reproductive system

Abortion   1
Adrenogenital Syndrome, 8
Cancer - breast, 41
Cancer - cervix, 43
Cancer - ovary, 49
Cancer - prostate, 51
Cancer - testis, 54
Cervicitis, 62
Cryptorchidism, 75
Dysmenorrhea, 89
Eclampsia - see Toxemia of Pregnancy, 277
Ectopic Pregnancy, 93
Endometriosis, 97
Endometritis, 98
Fibroadenoma - breast, 103
Fibrocystic disease - breast, 104
Fibroid, 105
Fibromyoma - see Fibroid, 105
Gonorrhea, 120
Leiomyoma - see Fibroid, 105
Mammary dysplasia - see Firocystic disease - breast, 104
Miscarriage - see Abortion, 1
Myoma - see Fibroid,   105
Ovarian Cysts, 196
Pelvic Inflammatory Disease (PID), 202
PMS - see Premenstural Syndrome, 221
Preeclampsia - see Toxemia of Pregnancy, 277
Pregnancy-induced Hypertension, 277

Premenstrual syndrome, 221
Prostatic Hyperplasia, 223
Prostatitis, 222
Salpingitis, 232
Syphilis, 256
Toxemia of Pregnancy, 277
Undescended testis - Cryptorchidism, 75
Vulvitis, 289

Respiratory system

Acquired Immuniodeficiency Syndrome, 4
AIDS - see Acquired Immuno Deficiency Syndrome, 4
Adult Respiratory Distress Syndrome, 9
Allergic rhinitis - see Hay Fever, 123
Anthracosilicosis - see Pneumoconiosis - Coal Worker's, 213
Anthracosis - see Pneumoconiosis - Coal Worker's, 213
ARDS - see Adult Respiratory Distress syndrome, 9
Aspergillosis - see Fungal infections, 111
Asthma - bronchial, 25
Atelectasis, 27
Beryllium disease - see Pneumoconiosis - Berylliosis, 212
Beryllium poisoning - see Pneumoconiosis - Berylliosis, 212
Blacklung disease - see Pneumoconiosis - Coal Worker's, 213
Bronchiectasis, 31
Bronchitis, 32
Bronchogenic Carcinoma, 47
Cancer - lung, 47
Coal miner's disease - see Pneumoconiosis, 213
Collapsed Lung - see Atelectasis, 27
Common cold, 68
Consumption - see Tuberculosis, 280
Cystic Fibrosis, 78
Emphysema, 95
Flu - see Influenza, 160
Fungal infections, 111
Grippe - see Influenza, 160
Hay fever, 123
Human Immunodeficiency Virus infection
    - see Acquired Immunodeficiency Syndrome, 4
Hyaline membrane disease
    - see Respiratory Distress Syndrome, 230
Infectious Mononucleosis, 157
Influenza, 160
Kissing disease - see Infectious Mononucleosis, 157
Laryngitis, 165
Lung abscess, 169